C000069844

The
4 Keys
to Health

Published by Snazell Publishing

Cromwell House
Wolseley Bridge
Stafford
Staffordshire
ST17 0XS
info@thepainkiller.co.uk

ISBN: 978-0-9931678-0-5

Paperback Edition 1st January 2015

The 4 Keys to Health

Nicky Snazell

Snazell Publishing

This book is dedicated to June D Brown, a dear close friend and reiki master, who sadly at the time of giving this book to the type setter, is close to death.

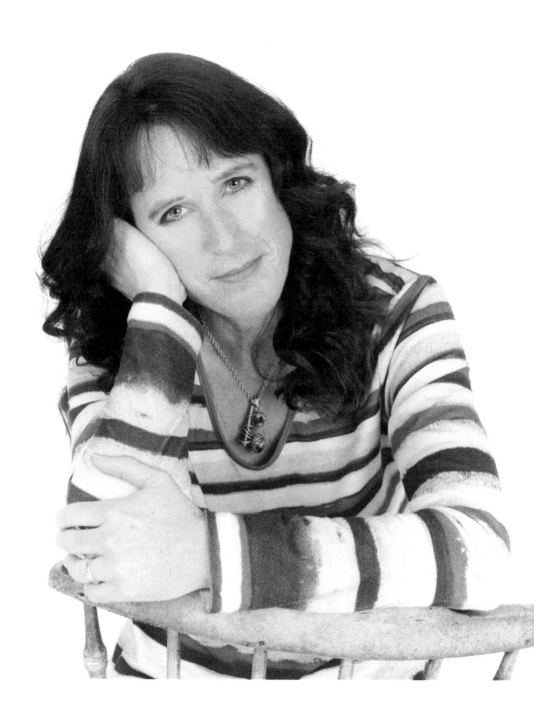

Praise for
The Four Keys To Health
by Nicky Snazell

A few years ago, I attended Nicky's clinic for a very painful 'frozen shoulder'. After many sessions of Nicky's considerable mix of technical treatments, I had considerable relief from the pain. This period of my life was beset with enormous pressures and anxieties, both professional and personal. Nicky taught me the importance of the effects of pain had on my life and helped me realise that through the addressing of that emotional pressure, the pain I was feeling would lift. Miraculously, as I took hold of the situations in my professional and personal life, the remaining discomfort just went. I got slimmer, fitter, and mind positive. The emotional effects of pain were diminished and I am now content, peaceful, and in 'my groove' in the next phase of my journey in this life, which is very exciting, with each new day unfolding pain free and mind easy. Thank you, Nicky.

– Barbara Herszenhorn, reiki master and children's book author.

Nicky is a unique individual; a multifaceted medical professional who is not afraid to draw on knowledge from a broad spectrum of specialties to aid her goal in understanding and treating pain as effectively as possible. Her understanding comes from both ends of the treatment spectrum; the cutting edge of research-based medical sciences and the more intuitive ancient, some may say, "sandals and candles" healing arts. In reality, Nicky places no preconceived boundaries on her knowledge or her willingness to learn, thus enabling her to develop the "real world" skills to help those in need around her. This book is the distillation of her life's work so far and encapsulates the learning and understanding from across this wide variety of sources. Spend some time in the company of Nicky Snazell and learn from her the keys to unlock your potential and to see a clearer way to helping yourself improve your own health, regardless of your current state.

– Jon Hobbs MSc MCSP FHEA
Consultant physiotherapist, acupuncture tutor, international lecturer.
Acupuncture Association of Chartered Physiotherapists Director.

An eye-opener of a book that will change the way you deal with pain forever and will set you on a new path. The "Pain Killer" – Nicky Snazell – will transform your life.

– Carol E Wyer, best-selling author of Grumpy Old Menopause.

I've had the privilege of working with Nicky Snazell at several Z Factor health seminars. She's a mesmerising speaker and her life work in pain treatment and management is always on the leading edge. Most of all, I've come to know Nicky's heart. Nobody cares more and wants to help you more than Nicky.

– John Lewis Parker, musician, mentor,
and international speaker and teacher on meditation.

This book is so important to grasp because one's good health depends on having healthy body cells.

– Professor Chan Gunn, clinical professor of anaesthesia,
consultant at the University of Washington, Seattle, and founder of IMS at
the Sports Medicine Centre at Calgary University, British Columbia.

Contents

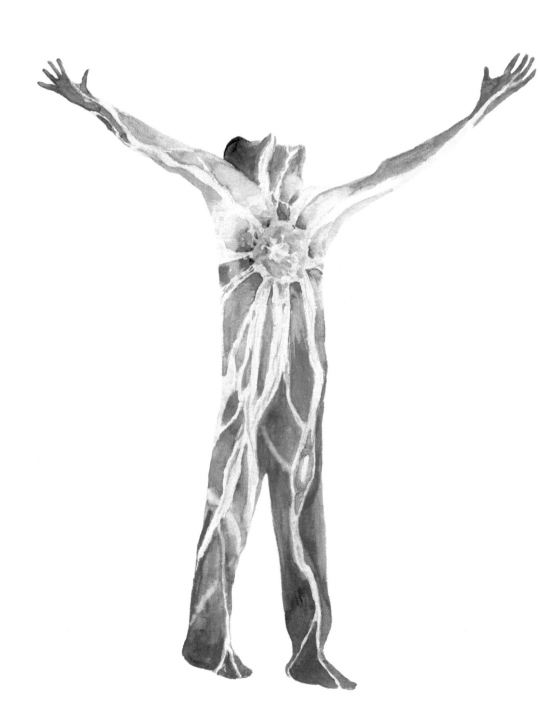

Introduction

Look to this day
for it is life
the very life of life
In its brief course lie all
the realities and truths of existence
the joy of growth
the splendor of action
the glory of power
For yesterday is but a memory
And tomorrow is only a vision
But today well lived
makes every yesterday a memory
of happiness
And every tomorrow a vision of hope
Look well, therefore, to this day!

– Ancient Sanskrit Poem

My name is Nicky Snazell and I am known to some as 'the pain killer'. After all, that's what I do: I kill pain, and I can kill yours too. I realise how important it is to free our bodies of pain so that we can enjoy our lives to the full, and I can help you to do exactly that. As the owner of a pain relief clinic in Staffordshire, I've got years and years of experience in treating pain and all of its causes, some of which we are frequently unaware of. So often I feel like I'm working in the illness industry and not the wellness industry, and I believe that we should focus more on the latter – by preventing health problems before we have to cure them.

I can get you to your optimal health for your age, no matter what your ability level. How? For one thing, I have studied health and pain for thirty years, researching how we as humans function at our best. Furthermore, this is backed up by the knowledge and skills I have gained by creating and working within my integrated medical practice, which has given me twenty-five years of hands-on experience and from which I've collected a long list of testimonials from satisfied customers who have managed to conquer their pain. They've done it, and now so can you.

I assume that if you're reading this book, you would like to know for certain that you can avoid a lot of unnecessary pain. Am I right? Then you've come to the right place. I want this book to be a practical resource that you can use and apply to your own health and your own life. After all, you are the author of your own life, so what chapter are you writing right now? You may have had no say in how your story started, but you have all the control in the world on what happens in the middle, as well as how many pages your novel contains. You have the power to control your own future health – you just need the knowledge and the skills to know how to do it. This is the information I'm going to give you in this book, and despite what you may have been led to believe, your pain is actually in your own hands.

I have spent my life searching for ways to treat pain, and I have travelled all over the world, meeting and learning from countless specialists and professionals during this quest of mine. Now, I want to pour all of that knowledge and all of my experience into this book, so that my methods can become your methods, and so that you can conquer your pain, allowing you to have a long, happy life. It sounds relatively simple, doesn't it? Well, it may be simpler than you think.

This book will discuss healing through an understanding of how neuroscience works, and I believe that this holds the keys to wellness, mental excellence, physical fitness, prosperity, relationship skills, society contribution and having a purpose to live – not to mention, of course, keeping out of pain. I like to imagine all of these things as breaking down into four main sections: the four keys of health, featuring mindset, nutrition and hydration, fitness, and lifestyle. You will be able to read about each of these four keys in the following chapters, and you can learn about the fifth key – how to deal with individual health problems – in my next book, *The Human Garage*. This will talk about what is lovingly nicknamed the 'clinic of last resort' by my patients.

Drawing from both modern medical technology and ancient healing wisdom, this book will guide you through your health journey, giving you the knowledge and the tools you need to create the best lifestyle for you. Say goodbye to pain and say hello to a fitter, healthier, happier you.

My Background

So, if you're considering taking my advice, you may want to know a little more about me and how I became interested in all things pain-related. Well, I was born in Rugby, but I moved to Staffordshire with my family when I was five. I currently live in the village of Little Haywood, with my pain relief clinic a five minute drive away; it is housed in a wonderful old building and is situated right on the edge of beautiful Cannock Chase. My clinic has treated more than 8,000 patients over the years, something which I'm very proud of. Many of these patients ask me why I'm based near Rugeley when I'm a world specialist – why aren't I in London or some other big city? The answer I always give to this question is that, simply, this is where my heart is. I love this area, and I love the building that houses my clinic. Like my patients, it has a rich history of its own, and I really believe that this beautiful setting is conducive to healing and becoming healthier and happier. This ambience wouldn't exist if it was set up in the middle of a heaving city. It's all about perception.

I loved books when I was little, and I read everything I could on a wide range of subjects, including science and how our bodies work. This early reading sparked my interest in health and life in general, and eventually this led to my focusing on human biology and psychology in a professional capacity. Even at a young age, I found that some things seemed obvious to me on a deep, intuitive level. For instance, I could sense when a person had knee pain or if they were grieving; it was something that just came to me, I couldn't help it. I soon learnt not to advertise these intuitions, as not everyone would understand or accept my skills. It was certainly not a common belief that things such as pain could be simply 'sensed'. Still, from then on, I had a clear understanding of suffering, and how the pain in a person's body could be affected by what was happening in their daily lives.

So, why did I choose this career path? Well, it is undeniable that our experiences shape us; they make us who we are and drive us on to achieve the things in life that give us – and our loved ones – more pleasure and less pain, wouldn't you agree?

I can think of one strong experience that framed my career choice, one that has been pivotal in bringing me here to write this book for you. This was watching my mother suffer from increasing and inexplicable back pain over several years, starting when I was in my teens. You know, that time in your life when things are black and white and when you lack buckets of experience to cope with the problems that life throws at you. We travelled to various doctors, surgeons and physical therapists, with the constant hope and the belief that the magic bullet would be out there. With endless patience, I sought out help, believing that someone must be able to give her relief; after all, wasn't that their job? As a patient, didn't my mother have a right to expect this?

The memories of fear, disappointment, and frustration – as well as the lack of knowledge at an important growing-up time – still haunt me. I had no tools in my tool box that could ease her pain. Can you relate to this? At this point, I was no closer to making a career choice. As far as I was concerned, modern medicine had let me down, and I had no desire to spend my life giving patients empty promises, with very little time actually allocated to their visits. As I said, I was a teenager, angry and wounded by society, and my belief at the time was that 'the system' had failed my mother.

Because of this, I initially chose to give medicine and pain a wide birth, instead deciding to undertake a science degree at university. This idea of a wide birth was short-lived, however, as I found a fascination for how biological systems worked, as well as being captivated by the complexity of life. I spent a lot of time in my third year writing up my research in the Queen Elizabeth Hospital library.

Then, one day, in the middle of my final year exams, a freak reaction to a routine medical procedure caused my left elbow to seize up to the point where I couldn't use my arm. This resulted in frequent and painful visits upstairs to the hospital physiotherapy department. During this time, I had one of those 'this is what I'm meant to be doing' epiphany moments and I came away with both a functioning arm and a career path in mind. Frustrated by the inability for physiotherapy to help with many different forms of pain, I studied as much as I could, searching continuously across a broad spectrum of subjects – both conventional and unconventional, Western and Eastern – and making sure I wasn't hemmed in by irrelevant rules and beliefs.

My only concerns were how I could learn to improve someone's health and how I could alleviate their suffering, two concepts which were soon interwoven into a single goal: health transformation. This has been my focus for years, and it is what this book is all about. I was by now intensely motivated to search for ways to alleviate all sorts of pain, without someone resorting to taking drugs for the rest of their life. I had a plan: I would marry specialist physical therapy techniques with psychology and healing, and I would find a cure for spinal pain. I would have a clinic with healers and surgeons working together, and I would find a synergy of treatments that would profoundly improve the quality of life for those who had previously been suffering. And, by and large, I've done it all.

For ten of those years, I managed hospital physiotherapy departments in the day, and my clinic in the evenings. Beyond treating, studying, and teaching, I also have the ever-exciting and demanding challenge of evolving a health business with my husband, which employs a wonderful team of friends. I have travelled all over the world to meet and learn from some of the top health gurus, having visited America, Canada, Italy, Switzerland, Korea, China, Malta, and many more places to expand my knowledge base. One of my most treasured gifts is a beautiful silver plaque, the first fellowship that Professor Gunn handed out, 'in recognition of extensive knowledge, outstanding contributions and expert teaching abilities in pain'. Professor Chan Gunn is a dear friend of mine and a brilliant world-renowned guru in pain relief himself, having spent years mapping out muscle activity using EMG (Electromyography) and having developed the plunger for use in IMS (Intramuscular Stimulation).

I am not stating all this to brag or to boast; I am simply telling you this to hopefully gain your trust and to try and convince you that reading this book is worthy of your time. I hope you agree with me, because if put into practice correctly, these pages are potentially life changing.

My Work Today

When it comes to describing who I am today, I find it a very difficult thing to do. This is because it depends on which hat I'm wearing on any particular day, which could be anything including: a biologist, a consultant physiotherapist, a pain lecturer, a pain treatment instructor to physiotherapists, GPs and consultants around the world, an international presenter, a writer on optimum health, an entrepreneur, the director/founder of painreliefclinic. co.uk, a director of MRT, and the founder/creator of nickysnazell.com. I generally find myself outside the normal rules and beliefs, because I take my knowledge from several different areas of medicine and healing, never ruling out any form of pain relief, whether it's the latest in medical science or an ancient tribal method, passed down through the generations. My life's journey – and all of the knowledge that I've gained – has led me to where I am now, and I'm delighted that I am able to teach others internationally on the subjects of pain and health.

Yes, I can call on my formal qualifications and subsequent specialist skills in chronic spinal pain, but now I've gone full circle and have returned to my earlier beliefs regarding pain and suffering: that the level of suffering is often the result of several factors, some of which the patient might not even be aware of. These can include what's going on in a person's life at the time, how stressed they are, what their beliefs are, how content they are with their life, and so on. All of these factors – and more – have as much impact on the degree of suffering as physical factors do (such as a fall or injury). This is what many people don't seem to realise, as they're always looking for external explanations for their pain instead of focusing on the bigger picture of their life, which we often have to look at when diagnosing and healing pain.

I strongly believe that interweaving modern medicine and technology with the ancient wisdom of intuitive healers is a powerful antidote to all kinds of unnecessary suffering in this modern world. Time and again I have witnessed my integrative approach gently soothe the suffering etched on my patients' faces.

An Integrative Approach to Health

So, what do I mean when I talk about integrative approaches? For instance, you may be wondering why I look at mindset (and why I've made it the first key and therefore the first chapter in this book) when I work with physical injuries. I firmly believe that if we get better at listening to the voices of our body, then we can heal the scars of trauma. In my experience, improving our understanding of the mind-body interaction within the treatment of disease leads to far greater success. I love the words, "Wisdom of the felt sense," and my interpretation of them is that we need to hone both the instinct of an animal and the intelligence of a human being. As humans, we have a tendency to translate pain into suffering – when they are actually two separate things – and so developing these innate skills can avoid unnecessary suffering.

Unfortunately, pain and ageing is a fact of life, but it is how we handle it that influences our quality of life, not our age or the pain itself. So, what has interweaving medicine, physical therapy and alternative therapies really achieved for me? I now understand how scientific facts, ancient shamanic knowledge, and the roles of both modern medicine and technology have enabled the best proven ideas to give an empowering combination that I can then use to heal my patients. This approach is an ever-changing and evolving one, as new ideas are developed around the world every day.

We speak of striving for 'good health', but what does this mean and how exactly do we measure it? I will share with you the tools you need to be able to better control your thoughts, put superior fuel in your body, and move in a healthy way for you, as well as how to look at your life and decide what support you need in terms of family, friends, your identity within society, the building you live in, and your environment in general.

Within my practice, I have created a unique model to activate, accentuate and evaluate an anti-ageing preventative cellular healing process for damaged joints. Yes, once a patient has agreed to work towards optimum health, we can speed up the healing of broken bones, arthritic joints, and prolapsed spinal discs. Helping people in this way is very life-enriching, rewarding work, and you can read more about these treatments in my next book, *The Human Garage*. The book you're reading now is all about how you can do your homework to prevent as many health problems as possible from arising.

So, what qualifies me to be able to help you? As a biologist, I have spent several years looking at how the environment affects our cells, so when I came to physical medicine, it was with a very different understanding of optimum health. For instance, I could see how the cells would change direction and shape with invisible signalling between them. I also studied evolution, seeing how intelligent creation drove the species development, and how it didn't just happen due to random occurrences. While I was fascinated by cells and biology in general, I didn't want to be a GP. I wanted to use everything I knew – including biology, but also things like psychology and physiotherapy – to be able to treat patients in my own way, without having to adhere to strict guidelines and time constraints that help no one.

I feel very strongly about the issues with time at doctors' practices and hospitals, whether it be too little time dedicated to patients or too much time spent on meetings, which inevitably leads to less patient care time. Actually, my belief that ward meetings took up too much patient care time was so strong at one point, that I risked getting struck off for unusual behaviour.

In my youthful days of working on a head injury unit, I quickly tired of lengthy team meetings, which could have been conducted in a much shorter time span. Here, everyone shared opinions about the patients' care, but I was so frustrated that no action ever seemed to be taken – we were just talking aimlessly whilst patients lay in beds needing urgent attention. I felt that I wasn't being listened to, so one day after covering hydrotherapy, I donned my full sub aqua gear and walked up the corridors to attend the meeting: I had the snorkel, the fins, the lot.

As it turned out, while I was in my gear, they *did* listen to my thoughts, and it was all going well until I caught the psychiatrist's coffee with a fin, and he got a wet lap. Scuba gear around hot beverages is apparently a no-go. Needless to say, my name was not on the following week's minutes, however, they did agree to reduce the number of meetings and push their thoughts into actions. The psychiatrist kept a worried eye on me, especially as I was promoted early on in my career to run an outpatients musculoskeletal unit, which had a pool! Because of this, I was nicknamed flipper.

Along the same lines, I was working at a local hospital when my boss at the time – knowing I was a biologist as well as a physiotherapist – asked me to remove some bats, which had managed to enter the orthopaedic ward. Well, of course, I was only too happy to help. I donned the gear – a black cape, two matchsticks and red lipstick – and dressed as Dracula, I rode a theatre trolley down to the ward. The bats left through the window unharmed, and although my boss caught me, he let me off with just a verbal warning – after all, the bat problem had been dealt with! Perhaps this is one of many reasons I now run my own clinic; my thinking was just a little too outside the box for them!

Avoiding Pain

So, I'm here to write about avoiding pain, which isn't something that most people want to think about, is it? But what's the opposite of pain? That's right: pleasure. We all do everything we can to avoid pain and seek pleasure, don't we? But do we always make conscious decisions to seek pleasure and avoid pain? Let's think about that. Is it possible that you make decisions that you perceive will give you pleasure when, in fact, it will ultimately give you pain? Yes, of course it is! We are all guilty of putting coins in the pain bank for long-term savings, rather than in the pleasure bank.

I have been puzzling over this one for many years while sitting in front of my patients. Recently, in preparation for The Z Factor – an annual health seminar run by Joseph McClendon III, where I give presentations – I asked my dear old friends, whom I've had the privilege of studying psychic/intuitive healing with for thirty years, about this. They responded with, "You have studied the pain behaviour of thousands of humans over the years, and still you are confused. Study *you*... listen to *your*self... ask yourself the question about all of *your* actions. Knowledge is inside us, not out there. Bring soul awareness, if you will. Bring mindfulness to your human thought processing when you make a decision about eating, working out, and so on. Get into a state of mind that is truthful about your actions."

When we bring into focus a higher awareness, we are checking our beliefs about what we see and feel. Our vision is very inaccurate, seeing only a tiny part of what is really there. If we see the colour red, we get the memory of what red means to us, making a meaning solely for us. Therefore, red is a belief. Higher awareness says that we are accessing memory data associated with this visual input in order to get hold of the belief. We run it through a semantic memory system, finding the belief and making it into a thought. Changing beliefs kills old habits.

What we need to realise is that we are controlled by social acceptance to do what everybody else does, and that we are all intensely manipulated by advertising. We are driven to believe what we see on TV and in the press. Drugs companies, food companies and drinks companies are not driven to provide the healthiest products they can, but to maximise their profits and serve their shareholders. The only person who can look after *you* is *you*, and if all you do is follow everyone else, you are doing no better than a lemming who blindly follows the rest of the lemmings off a cliff (for any children reading this, my friend Jon Hobbs has just informed me that this was a Walt Disney idea and that lemmings don't actually do this). Anyway, when we think of pain, we need to realise that many causes of pain are self-inflicted and can be easily avoided. So, why do people choose the self-destruct button, over and over again? This is the fundamental question about pain, and one which needs to be answered. For many, pain is a choice.

Every day, I sit in front of gentle folks who are overweight, eating rubbish and not exercising. For example, Mr Smith has knee arthritis, and is 'too short for his weight'. He came to see me as he's scared of having new prosthetic knee joints, something which is relatively common. Now, I must be honest – I'm a little too short for my weight, too. Hands up those of you who would like to be taller for your weight! My trouble can be that I eat a few too many calories, and why do I do this? Pleasure. Specifically, short-term pleasure. "Just a little more fruit… it won't hurt, will it?"

Now, let's think about my arthritic friend, sitting in my office, using up two chairs to do so. Arthritis is the leading cause of disability and has been for fifteen years. It is a problem that affects millions of people and which causes massive pain and a huge loss in quality of life. Compared to non-sufferers, those with arthritis experience three times as much lost work due to having time off. Arthritis means big pain. Obesity doubles the risk of arthritis. Lack of exercise also doubles the risk. Therefore, there are some simple things we can do to reduce our chances of suffering from arthritis, and this can be said for most diseases. We just need to educate ourselves as to what these preventative measures actually are.

As I've mentioned, pain isn't always the result of something physical, such as a fall or recent injury. We can actually trap pain into places in our body from things such as hidden beliefs, stress, fear, and tragic memories. Have you got any pain in your body that could relate to something in your past? It's more common than you might think, and once you've identified the source of this pain, it is much easier to start the healing process.

The Statistics of Pain

One of the main questions I ask myself is: why do so many of us choose pain? The numbers are just staggering. For example, more than 632 million people worldwide suffer from lower back pain – a leading cause of disability – and the sad thing is, people are choosing this pain instead of doing something about it. In the UK today, 900,000 people are housebound, and often bedridden, with no help and no hope of getting better. We are supposedly a wealthy country with a healthy lifestyle, so how can this be?

According to the Institute of Medicine, one-third of all Americans (that's approximately 100 million adults) suffer from chronic pain of some sort, which exceeds the number of people who are affected by heart disease, diabetes and cancer combined. The economic costs of medical care and loss of productivity total more than $550 billion annually. It is an incredible sum of money, and it simply doesn't have to be this way.

Personally, I have spent thirty years studying how we can improve the ways our cells function, as well as the way we move and walk, our pain avoidance, and the intricate communication system between our minds and our bodies. We have come a long way in our understanding of illness, from dissecting diseased tissue to epigenetics, which looks at how a healthy lifestyle controls the timing of when our genes are switched on and off. Why is it then, that with all of this knowledge, we still have a growing epidemic of back pain and general musculoskeletal problems? In the UK, more than 10 million souls go to their doctor with this kind of complaint every year, and with obesity on the rise, the numbers keep going up.

As I've said before, I strongly believe that integrative medicine is the way forward, combining the most potent aspects of medicine and complementary therapies. This combination doesn't always happen, though. Time and again I have seen cracks appear in patients' recovery when communication between professionals breaks down. This is sad because there is rarely just one cause and one solution to joint pain; teasing out the main problems and matching a unique treatment approach is key to giving someone their life back, and it is unfortunate that a lot of health professionals don't regard pain in this way.

In 2013, Simply Health conducted a survey of 1000 people living in the UK, aged between twenty-five and sixty-five, and found that 7 out of 10 people endured lower back pain, making it the nation's number one physical problem. It was interesting to see that out of these sufferers, 89% were very reluctant to seek help from physiotherapists, which in my opinion is fuelled by new NHS constraints on time and treatment modalities. It was also found that 40% of women felt old before their time due to multiple joint pains, and 28% were also depressed and frustrated by these problems. Men, on the whole, were less troubled by joint pain: 1 in 5 had knee pain, compared to 1 in 3 ladies, and only 25% felt older due to joint pains, with 23% feeling depressed about their situation.

Three quarters of the British public did not seek help from private physiotherapists, wrongly believing that their GP had to refer them. This lack of knowledge about their treatment options means that painkillers are still the most common way of dealing with back pain, despite us knowing the dangers of long-term use, which can include heart attacks, strokes, and high blood pressure. It is a sad fact that more than a third of Britons who suffer aches and pains believe they are just an inevitable part of ageing and that the only treatment is drugs. There are so many other options available to you.

We have a nation suffering when, with a little bit of awareness, a lot of these problems could be avoided. So, I continue to ask myself: why do so many of us choose pain? It is my intention to educate as many people as possible about their options, so hopefully we can bring the number of suffering Britons down.

What Pain Means

This brings us onto the question: what is pain? Many people view pain as being a bad thing in itself, but actually, it is nature's warning system, meant to protect us. When someone brings us bad news, we don't shoot the messenger, do we? Instead, we listen to what the messenger has to say, and then we go and find the *real* cause of the problem. It is exactly the same thing when it comes to pain: Mr Pain is only trying to warn us that there is a problem, and it is up to us to take his advice and seek out the true reason behind that pain – where is Mr Pain coming from? And why? This is what we have to find out.

Unfortunately, nature's warning system can so easily become a nightmare. Lasting pain can be caused by deficiencies and excesses in your mind, body, and diet. The secret to conquering pain is to find out what you have too much or too little of. It's all about balance, and any disruption in the delicate balance of your body can be a strong contender for the root cause of your painful life.

As we age, we need to put more care into our diet, our supplementation, our exercise, and our workload. It sounds simple, but many of us fail to even acknowledge that we have to change the way we use our bodies as we get older. As we age, naturally occurring enzymes are fewer, inflammation is greater, and the change from fibrinogen to inflexible scar tissue becomes much more extensive. Therefore, long-term solutions for pain need to address our ongoing biochemical changes.

I have two kinds of patients that come to my clinic: those who want a quick fix with no effort on their part or change in their lifestyle, and those who want a more permanent solution and actually want to make an investment in their future health. Long-term solutions can only be met by concentrating on the root cause, not by simply focusing on the symptoms alone.

How much we feel pain is governed by our beliefs and moods, as our joint psychology/biology (physiology) affects every cell in our body. What we don't know about pain will hurt us, but the body is always attempting to regulate pain impulses and to heal. With improved knowledge, we can work with – rather than against – this process and, in turn, feel less pain.

How Pain Works

So, how does pain work? We have a myriad of tiny receptors inside us – sensing touch, pressure, temperature, and pain – which pass information to our sensory nerves. These pain impulses travel up the dorsal horn of the spinal cord, and here is where you get your first chance to reduce your pain level - at the pain gate. If pain gets through the gate, it heads onto the thalamus, which acts like a router and – simply speaking – makes three 'phone calls', one to the sensory cortex (which interprets the nature of the pain), one to the mammalian amygdala (which assesses the level of fear, is the emotional centre, and which decides if the body needs to shut down digestion, cell division, circulation etc.), and one to the cortex (which is in charge of the human decision-making process).

Hence our minds really do decide, like a panel of judges, how much pain is appropriate for us to experience at any one time. Pain is then translated into how much we hurt. If we return to the gating mechanism, you can close the gate at the pain's entry point into the brain by doing several things. While we will explore these concepts in more depth in the individual chapters, they can include: having a massage, getting the right amount and the right type of sleep, undergoing acupuncture, eating nutritious food and making correct use of supplements, going to reiki and meditation sessions, evaluating your lifestyle, understanding your natural biorhythms, taking part in regular exercise, getting your posture right, using a TENS device, undergoing hypnosis, drinking plenty of water, doing breathing exercises, and making sure you get enough laughter into every day.

The Different Types of Pain

What are the different types of pain? Acute pain is when a patient has an accident or injury and the nociceptors (pain receptors) trigger an alarm impulse. This is useful pain – it's protective and necessary for survival. Chronic pain is when the signal has stopped serving a useful purpose. Pain travels through nerves, and these can be damaged due to repeated trauma or poor posture resulting in compression, however brief this may be.

Limbs are just an extension of your spine. When we were a ball of cells developing in the womb, we had cells dedicated to specific zones, such as the skin cells (dermatomes), the muscle cells (myotomes), and the organs (sclerotomes). These flow out from the spine to the limbs and are numbered according to the spinal segments to which they belong. Often, therefore, painful chronic problems will not switch off because a nerve is faulty, for example, with tennis elbow, plantar fasciitis, whiplash, and sciatica.

Poor posture, repeated injury, and wear and tear of the spine (spondylosis) can all cause the phenomenon of neuropathic pain. This is when the nerve becomes super-sensitive, which leads to false pain stimuli, as well as palpable muscle contractures and chronic degenerative tendonitis/tenosynovitis (where muscle attaches to the bone via the tendon). We feel pain long after the cause has happened. Unhelpful, unpleasant pain.

Of course, everyone has a reasonable idea that they need to exercise and eat healthily and have purposeful thoughts to do this, but you don't always do it, do you? You procrastinate. "I'll start tomorrow… I don't have the time… It's not my responsibility… I'm far too busy… I don't believe things will get better… I can't make a difference, not me, not just one person out of billions… I have more important priorities…" The excuses go on. What you have to remember is that, actually, your health is your number one priority, and nothing should come before it. If you want to have a happier, longer, pain-free life, where you can be around for your family and friends, you need to put your own health right at the top of your list. Everything else comes after.

I must confess: I've been in your shoes, many times, and yes, it's a constant battle. Remember how I felt about my mother? My endless anger and disappointment? Hating the fact that no one could do anything to help her? Well, she's conquered her problem now. In fact, she hasn't had it for about thirty-five years.

I strongly believe that integrative medicine is the way forward, combining the most potent aspects of modern medical practises and complementary therapies. My interest in ancient medicine and wisdom has taken me around the world, meeting shamans and healers who still use the ways of their ancestors. I also believe in – and use – modern technology (such as the magnetic resonance MRT machine we have at the clinic), and can I just ask: where does it say that I can't use both in my treatment of people and their pain? I gather techniques from all of these various types of healing, and I think that we should all be more open to the different ways in which we can help our bodies and, therefore, help ourselves. There is more that you can do – without the help of a doctor or a pill – than you may realise. In fact, there is a whole host of things you can put into practise to give yourself a longer, healthier life. And who wouldn't want that?

With my background, I am very aware of the power of the mind and I feel privileged to be in the driving seat of the physical medicine of tomorrow. I strongly believe that analysing any block to a patient (in terms of pain) and getting the healing results they want is incredibly important. In keeping accurate records and applying both an intuitive and scientific approach to health, we will be able to experience a broader understanding, something which will pave the way forward in terms of healing for future generations.

Looking At Your Own Pain

OK, this is something you can do right now. Stand up! If you're wearing trousers, roll them up to your knees, and take a look. Do you have varicose veins? What about the texture of your skin? Is it dry and tight, or soft and supple? Is it cold or hot to the touch? What do any of these things tell you? Well, varicose veins, dry skin or skin that is cold to the touch could all mean there is a problem back at the spine. This is just one example of how we always need to look at the bigger picture of our bodies.

Let's use an analogy. Imagine that your car headlight keeps flickering and that after a while, of course, the bulb eventually blows. So, you go to change the bulb. Then, that one keeps flickering and eventually blows as well. Now, most people would realise that if two bulbs have blown, then maybe the problem is not the bulb. Sure enough, when you check, you find that there's some bad wiring back at the fuse box. The body is just the same: a problem at the spine can have an effect elsewhere, such as dry skin, varicose veins, and coldness.

So, I want to get you thinking about which aspects of your life are healthy right now and which areas require urgent attention to prevent illness. If we take this one stage further and imagine the deterioration in health over a normal lifetime, then what we tend to see in the UK is a long, slow decline as we get older. Live short, die long. You may not know this, but the way you live actually accelerates the good or bad changes in your cells and in the way your genes are activated. We need to turn it around, living longer and dying shorter.

We all tell ourselves a story – I know I do – for every single injury or operation we have, and I have to be careful how I replay my story. This is because memory is fluid; every time we recall something, we mould a new version of it, and that is what our body remembers. We'll talk about this more in my mindset chapter.

Getting Over the First Hurdle

One of my memories that always conjures up nervous feelings is that of having to present in Vancouver. In the early days of my career I used to dread public speaking, that is, until I discovered mind NLP (Neuro-Linguistic Programming) techniques. Anyway, on one of my many trips around the world to study pain (the elusive devil), I was asked to work on and present a business plan – a vision of pain relief training in the future – in Vancouver. Professor Gunn was in charge (he of IMS plunger fame) and he had told me to arrive in plenty of time so I could have a slap-up meal the night before to chill out. So, on my arrival I was squeezed into a silk dress and supporting tights (as Madame was supposed to look very slim), which didn't impress me much as I had my thoughts channelled into a yummy supper after a long flight. When I entered the room, I found myself facing a whole host of fascinating people, from TV presenters to eminent professors and movie stars. It all looked like great fun, and I was most definitely ready to relax after all the travelling I'd done to get there.

We'd just sat down and I was about to start enjoying myself when my husband (who was then my bit of stuff) turned to me and said, "Don't pee your pants… but you're on the menu, as the European speaker, along with a smattering of some of the top surgeons from around the world." To say this came as a bit of a shock would be an understatement, and I saw Professor Gunn smile at me from across the room as my face drained of colour, my skin now matching the plain white linen cloths on the table. The people around me were plugging in laptops and checking sound systems, and the nerves had most certainly kicked in. It was at this point that my hubby told me, "we need to prepare", as if there wasn't currently a huge problem I had to face within the next few minutes. Needless to say, this irritated me slightly, as my mind was definitely not in the right place! So, with no warning and no notice, we scribbled a few words down on a napkin and I somehow found the strength to stride to the front of the room, even if I did look like a hedgehog which was just about to cross a busy motorway.

In the end, I had nothing to worry about; it went well and my words received a positive response from the audience. In fact, this singular event helped to improve my confidence in public speaking to an amazing degree. I just had to get over that first hurdle, which is what you need to do in order to start on your path to a pain-free life. Taking those first few steps towards a healthier existence can be scary, but they'll be more than worth it in the end. After my speech, I cornered Professor Gunn and he calmly informed me that it was a test. He needed someone who would speak from the heart, and that is exactly what I did. This, therefore, is the napkin version of my book – it is written straight from my heart, and I hope that you enjoy it and find it as useful as my Vancouver audience found my speech.

My aim is to continue to change people's lives in a really meaningful way, God willing, and for my methods to continue long after I've gone. What I'm really interested in is completely transforming the way that people look at their health and fitness, which in turn, transforms their lives. This is why I use a butterfly as the logo for my pain relief clinic, as the journey from a caterpillar into a fully-fledged butterfly is much the same as the journey my own patients go through. The butterfly itself is a symbol of transformation, and it represents the ability to change from one state to another, or in my patients' cases, from one lifestyle to another – from one burdened by pain, to one free of it.

I would like you to think about who you really are. What drives your life? What is most important to you? Have you written a life plan? You're probably planning on being around for a long time, and you may have a whole host of plans for your retirement. This is great, but you can't plan ahead without looking at – and evaluating – how your life is right now. The more you put off changing your lifestyle for the better, the less chance you'll get to do all of these amazing things you're planning for when you're older. It sounds scary, yes, but when you look at the figures, you may decide to start changing your life *now*. Studies in the USA have shown that students who write life plans are often much more successful in later life, showing how important it is to be prepared.

Getting To Retirement Age

Let's consider some facts, by again looking to the USA and their statistics on lifestyle at retirement age. Now, I want you to imagine that you're at a party with all your friends. Out of all of these people, how many do you think will still be alive at retirement age? How many will be flat broke? How many will be wealthy enough to help others? If we look at the American statistics here (which will be similar to our own in the UK), the answers to these questions may surprise you. Out of 100 American citizens with social security, only one would be wealthy at retirement age. Four would be financially secure. Five would still have to work in order to afford their lifestyle. Fifty-four would be completely broke, and thirty-six would be dead. Only 5% would be able to live healthy lives at this point. Now, imagine you're looking around at your friends at the party again. Only 5% of these people will be able to support themselves enough to live healthily at retirement age. This is why we need a life plan, and this is why we really need to think about where our lives are going.

With that in mind, how old do you think your kids will live to? And does it matter where in the world they live? Unfortunately, according to the CIA File (October 2014), the average life expectancy of children who are born now is not as good as you might think (especially with some scientists estimating that all of us will soon be living into our hundreds). Broken down by country, people born in Monaco today will have an average life expectancy of 89.57 years. This is at the top of the table. Here in the UK, it is 80.42 years. In the USA, 79.56 years. Then, right at the bottom of the table, we have South Africa: children being born there today will have a life expectancy of just 40.96 years. This sounds shocking, but it is something that – here in the UK – we have the power to change ourselves, by transforming the way we think, what we eat, how we move, and what kind of lifestyle we choose to have.

That's right – it's a choice. We can choose to prove those figures wrong and live long, healthy lives, or we can do nothing, and watch as our life spans get shorter and shorter. It's a decision we can actively make for ourselves, and it's a decision that we shouldn't have to spend too long contemplating. If we want to have longer lives, we have to start changing *now*.

Traffic Light Approach to Health

At my clinic, I always ask my patients to fill in a questionnaire about their current health, and their answers are incredibly useful in letting me see where they need to improve their mindset, their nutrition, their fitness and their lifestyle. I call it the traffic light approach to health because we analyse these areas by saying whether the patient is green (good), amber (room for improvement) or red (poor). These are your fitness keys, and they will tell you where you need to improve. With this in mind, I have developed four questionnaires – one for each key – and have placed them in the appendix of this book. If you want to get the most out of this book, I urge you to complete the questionnaire at the start of each chapter, and again after you've absorbed the knowledge and implemented some of my suggested changes into your life. Soon, you should start to see your traffic light scores changing from red or amber to green on all counts. When this happens, you are likely to be at your optimal health for your age, which means you'll be giving yourself the best possible chance if a disease or injury should occur.

So, to those therapists and doctors who want to go beyond their specific training and look at the synergy of everything they know in order to create their own map, here is mine.

If you don't want to commit to a new, healthy you, then now is probably a good time to leave. If, however, you desire to work towards a healthy, fit, pain-free body, here we go. It's time to take your health into your own hands and get rid of all the pain that has been holding you back.

We begin by looking at our mindset.

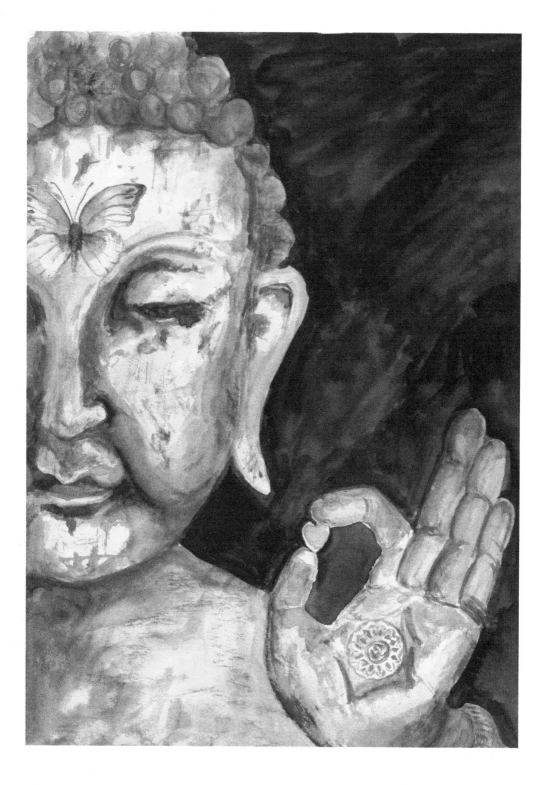

Mindset

You Can Be Whatever You Want To Be

There is inside you
all of the potential to be whatever
you want to be –
all of the energy to do whatever
you want to do.
Imagine yourself as you would like to be,
doing what you want to do,
and each day, take one step
toward your dream.
And though at times it may seem too
difficult to continue,
hold on to your dream.
One morning you will awake to find
that you are the person
you dreamed of –
doing what you wanted to do –
simply because you had the courage
to believe in your potential
and to hold on to your dream.

– Donna Levine

Before you read this chapter, please go to page 247 of the appendix and complete the traffic light questionnaire for mindset.

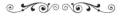

How to Drive Our Mind

Why our thoughts affect our health and life

And so we start our journey of health transformation by looking carefully at our mindset.

"A new philosophy, a way of life, is not given for nothing. It has to be paid for dearly and only acquired with much patience and great effort." – Fyodor Dostoyevsky.

This was true in Dostoyevsky's time, and it is very much still true today. If you are looking to transform your health in order to live the happiest, longest life you possibly can, then you need to put the effort in. The good news is that you've already made the first step by identifying your desire to get healthier, and you've even now made the second step by reading this book. This is clearly something that you want, so are you ready to put the work in?

This chapter is all about giving you the knowledge and the tools you need in order to seek out the help you require, giving you the correct keys to open the doors in your mind and finding yourself thinking healthier thoughts.

With all of the modern day technology we have available at our fingertips – the many screens we use throughout the day, constantly being attached to our phones, relying on electronics for most of our daily activities – we've lost something of ourselves. We've become very alien to what we're actually capable of doing, of the potential that our bodies and our minds have. Contrary to popular belief, magic does happen – it's just that we have to open our minds up to the possibility of it happening. People with certain beliefs and with an understanding of their own energy can not only help to heal themselves, but can also help to heal others. It's all about getting in the correct mindset.

The Power of the Mind

My own interest in the power of the mind began in my late teens and early twenties, when I was introduced to the subject through Wicca. Wiccans believe that you can use the power of the mind to both heal yourself and send healing to people over a distance. They use meditation and relaxation techniques to get into the right state of mind, and during this ritual they can actually change their brainwaves and focus on their ancient gifts, something that people today have forgotten all about. They can actually drive their own minds. This distant healing has been tested in studies – for example, in China they have recorded instances of people with cancer, whose tumours actually shrank while people were praying over them.

Your own mindset is paramount to all aspects of your health. Without a positive, long-term commitment to health, you will not eat and drink well, you will not make sure that you get regular and adequate exercise, you will not actively seek a positive lifestyle, and you will not be able to control your stress. Without first getting your head in the right place, how can you expect to make all of these changes to your life? As with any life decision, you have to make sure you are in the right mindset, and that you're making these changes for the right reasons. If you're trying to please someone else or if you're only doing it to get a nagging family member off your back, you're more than likely not going to stick with it. If you're doing it for you, and because *you* want to have a longer and healthier life, then you *will* be able to stick with it.

In fact, if you are unfulfilled or feel unloved, you may exaggerate or even manufacture health problems in order to gain attention. For example, you may be in pain, but you may not necessarily want to lose that pain. Pain is your path towards attention and love, whether it be from family, friends, or your therapist. Without your pain, you may be afraid that no one will notice you. For you, pain is your route to significance. If this is the case, you can see why we first need to change your mindset before you can even begin to start changing your eating or exercise habits. If you don't want the pain to go away, it won't. You have to *want* this for yourself.

Because of this, we need to establish that it is your own decision to get healthy. Once you get to your optimal health, you will be more likely to have the tools to beat any health problem or illness that comes your way, but you need to remember that preventative medicine is your own responsibility, not your doctor's. Learning about the four keys to health – and putting them into practise – will help you to be the best you can be, and will get you in good stead for when any health problems do come along. By first preparing your mind, you can then prepare your body.

Over the years, I have come to realise that about 70% of suffering is linked to emotional baggage, which destroys any enjoyment of life. Pain does not equate to the same amount of suffering, and working out the cause of the suffering is like finding the tuft of wool you need from a woven ball. Once you find it and pull it out, everything unravels beautifully and you can begin to knit a new you.

You may not realise that the marriage between your unconscious and your conscious is not always a happy one. This is because the former reacts coldly to your chattering thoughts. I will give you an introduction to meditation so you can start – like with the ball of wool – to unravel your chattering mind. I will also give you some everyday tapping techniques to focus your mind on positive thoughts.

I will expand on how what you think about yourself affects your actions – and hence your future – later on in the chapter. For those of you who have heard of 'The Secret', I will be touching upon the science behind it, as well as NLP (Neuro-Linguistic Programming), the way your brain is wired, and how you can use the essence of it for your own benefit.

Preventing Illness with the Mind

At university, I was taught all about illness. Alternative medicine, however, taught me about preventing illness by studying healthy, happy people, and by asking them how they achieved their optimum health. Time and again the key ingredient was hopeful, optimistic, and proactive thoughts; these individuals would actively seek out and pursue wellbeing in appropriate ways to achieve long, healthy lives, and they possessed an excellent internal dialogue and communication skills with others. When asked how they achieved this, on the whole it would be through practise, being taught by parents or friends, or through disciplined meditation.

Quoted in Deepak Chopra's book *Perfect Health*, Dr Keith Wallace headed up some research which showed that the biological markers of ageing can actually be slowed down with meditation. 84 meditators were used in the study, with an average age of fifty-three, and they were split into two groups: one with participants who had been meditating for under five years, and the other with meditators of five years and over. The short-term meditators were five years younger than their chronological age, with the long-term meditators being an astounding twelve years younger than their chronological age. On top of this, Dr Jay Glaser found that older meditators had as much of the anti-ageing hormone DHEA as non-meditators who were five to ten years younger (Chopra, 1991).

Do You Know How To Listen?

I think you would agree that intuitive listening is a skill most of us could improve upon, and being able to communicate our feelings to each other (as well as to ourselves) is necessary to achieving both health and happiness. If we feel listened to and understood, we feel cherished. In the same way, so do our trillions of cells.

Our thoughts are interpreted as good or bad by our brain. This creates a cascade of neurotransmitters and also fires off the adrenal gland to release 'fight or flight' chemicals according to the degree of fear. These neuropeptides are secreted not only in the brain but in every cell in the body, creating a direct impact on the immune system, controlling cellular inflammation and abnormal growth.

Many drugs – including those used for arthritis – are targeted at the end point of this cascade. However, I want you to go back to the beginning and change your thoughts to elicit a different emotional and chemical response. Our fragile immune system is very sensitive, being very self-destructive when there is negative input involved, and the consciousness that creates new cells is so often locked in the past. Our cellular membranes have an energy matrix – with good or bad memories embedded within it – which affects the health of the cell. It is amazing that our white cells can carry memories of previous, emotionally-charged events in our lives, and when a similar chain of events fire off the same thoughts, we get a huge army of white cells, which can lead to an inflammatory attack or infection within 24 to 48 hours of having these thoughts.

This is why I always ask my patients what was happening in their life at the time of a diagnosis (say, of rheumatoid arthritis or cancer). Furthermore, I ask what happened to their genetic predecessors: these will still have an impact on your health as their memories are also encoded in your cells. The way we are wired is incredible; if your earlier family members – great grandparents or grandparents, for instance – drowned, or were scared of spiders, then the fear and immune response will be so much stronger to this stimuli in your own body.

So, we now know that it is important to avoid fearful or negative thoughts. To illustrate this, I recently came across an interesting yet little-known piece of research (by David McIowen), whereby effects of certain stimuli on the immune system were measured. By using medical students – and samples of their salivary glands – each was asked to watch an hour of a programme on either gardening, war, or Mother Teresa, and the impact on the immune system was clear. War had a harmful effect, Mother Teresa generated a very positive effect, and with the more neutral gardening, there was no change.

This study shows that it is a good idea to reduce the impact of unpleasant media that can stress the central nervous system (CNS).

Now I want to tell you about my favourite listening exercise for improving relationships, and if you take it seriously, this can be life changing. My team did this recently during our weekly teaching sessions, which we do to make sure we are up to speed with our communication skills.

What you have to do is sit down with a friend or partner and role play at being their therapist. You will need to draw out a timetable of daily activities, in thirty minute chunks. Then, write the activities underneath, such as '8 a.m. drive to work for 30 minutes', 'work at computer for an hour' and so on. Listen carefully to the words they use, as well as their body language when they're talking about each activity, and then write down a key emotion beneath that activity. Your partner needs to write down their actual emotion, and then you can compare notes afterwards. Now, be honest, and put a score down of how well you listened, before swapping over. You can repeat this a week later to see if your listening has improved. Many little exercises like this can help to improve our listening and communication skills, and thus improve our mindset.

What memories of your life do your cells hold? Look back at the amount of time you've felt content and then increase it, either by your attitude or by your activities, in order to make your life more purposeful and happy. Stop as soon as you have a negative thought, and when you have a positive one, hang on for at least fifteen seconds. This will help to re-programme your cells, allowing you to be the architect of the new you. Change your consciousness, change your cells, change your life.

Every day, I get the privilege of changing lives by creating tailor-made programmes that nurture the immune system. Being able to create the right mind state and brain wave pattern is a crucial step towards being in optimum health. Preventative medicine, in the form of changing your thoughts, takes time, patience, and a lot of hard work. It doesn't mean that we escape illness and death, but it does mean that we've simply done the best we can to reduce our suffering.

A quote from Doctor Zhivago is appropriate here: "The great majority of us are required to live a life of constant systematic duplicity. Your health is bound to be affected if, day after day, you say the opposite of what you feel, if you grovel before what you dislike and rejoice at what brings you nothing but misfortune. Our nervous system isn't just a fiction, it's part of our physical body, and our soul exists in space and is inside us, like the teeth in our mouth. It can't be forever violated with impunity."

Your life's destiny is not what happens to you, instead it is what you do and the decisions you make. You cannot control the outside environment – you can't change the heatwaves, rains, floods, and snow that our climate experiences. You can't change the world economy, either, or how your country is doing financially. You can, however, control your inside environment: what you do, what you learn, and what you do with your knowledge. This is your power.

Many of today's powerful people were not born privileged in terms of wealth or family. They may not have had a great start in life, but they made conscious decisions to be all they could be, and not to accept anything less. They shaped their destiny from within, and so can you. You see, exceptional people never stop seeking new ways to learn, and that is exactly what you are doing now by reading this book.

I have had the honour of studying with – and, on occasion, presenting with – such people. These individuals have inspired literally millions through their seminars and books, and they have been sought out by Kings, Presidents, and movie stars. Each of these people have endured life changing experiences, which in part have guided their chosen life paths.

Changing the Way You Think

I have come into contact with many patients over the years who have had to change the way they think about their bodies and their health. One such case featured a man, Joseph, caring for his mother. In 1998, Joseph's mother was diagnosed with intestinal cancer, and her doctors gave her just two months to live. This is terrible news for any son to hear, but through his 'ultimate performance' training, Joseph knew that if his mother was told this, she would almost certainly die within the two months. She would believe her diagnosis, and not thinking there was any hope, her body would listen to her mind and begin to shut down. Because of this, he asked the doctors not to tell her. Instead, he got her to change her lifestyle, her eating habits, and – most importantly for her – her mindset. She didn't die within two months. She didn't even die within twelve months. Joseph's mother lived for another eleven and a half healthy years.

This is so important, that I will say it again: his mother lived more than *eleven years longer* than her doctors gave her by changing her lifestyle, eating habits and mindset. What value would you place on such wisdom? This experience resulted in Joseph McClendon redirecting and recharging his focus to health and wellbeing, researching what the main ingredients are to a healthy life, and he now runs The Z Factor, an annual event that I often present at myself.

Stress Management

All of us are becoming more aware of stress and its dangers, and where stress is lurking, so is fear. Fear and pain are sisters; enduring unremitting stress can overwhelm our immune systems, leaving us open to cellular disasters like cancer. This is why we need to learn how to deal with stress and bring awareness to what it is doing to us on both an emotional and physical level.

In this day and age, we are constantly bombarded with… well, everything. Buying stuff, cleaning stuff, fixing stuff, storing stuff, just having stuff and paying people to maintain it… you name it, we have to deal with it. We are sheep, and we simply must keep up with the Joneses.

The way most of us deal with stress is by choosing things and activities that give us immediate gratification – chocolate, drink, smoking, sex… does this sound familiar? How about changing your reactions to stress and doing some exercise? Talking to loved ones? Getting a massage? Or just some good food, in moderation? Doesn't that sound better than diabetes, cancer, depression, an early death or slow, painful rot? This is what stress does to us, and it's what it will continue to do to us if we react to it by choosing things that are bad for us.

If we spend eight hours a day feeling stressed, our cells cannot divide properly. Our gut cannot digest, our muscles don't work properly, and our immune system starts to shut down. Our brainwaves aren't easily able to reach a relaxed state, and our happiness is long gone.

We can test whether we're stressed or not in many ways, and one of which is a small device called the HeartMath. You put your thumb on this instrument, and the light turns red when you are stressed. Patrick Holford first introduced me to this clever device when I was up on stage, and when my reading showed burnout, he suggested that I read his book on stress and fatigue!

I actually took this to my presentation at Joseph McClendon's Z Factor in Switzerland, and most people in the audience were red. It's shocking, really, as most of the time, we wouldn't even know that we were particularly stressed – at least, no more than usual. I wired my co-star John Parker (our meditation guru) up to this during my talk and asked him to go into a meditative state. With the help of the HeartMath, I could demonstrate how his brain waves altered and how his heart rate variation got better and his breathing slowed. Coming out of fight or flight means that we can heal, sleep, and grow cells.

There are many different techniques for reducing stress if you're suffering from insomnia. For example, counselling can be combined with a form of biofeedback before going to bed to reduce beta activity that keeps you awake. Focus on slowing down your breathing and deepening it using HeartMath. Brainwaves must be correct to heal, relax, digest, divide cells, and so on. Meditative CDs can also help reduce stress and send you off to a peaceful sleep. Alpha waves are a nice mind state to treat and heal patients in, while gamma and theta are for deeply relaxing, healing, meditating, and dreaming.

Dealing With Stress Evoked By Living with Chronic Pain

Chronic pain is a very uncomfortable and worrisome experience. Those who live with it, perhaps after suffering injuries or perhaps through living with a condition like arthritis, worry about flare-ups every day.

A new health breakthrough states that avoiding stress is key for pain relief. This particular study wanted to measure specific indicators that are related to stress, in 16 patients with chronic back pain and in 18 healthy people. The indicators they used were cortisol levels (also known as the 'stress hormone'), people's perception of their own pain, the size of their hippocampus (the brain region involved in pain and anxiety), and how the brain responds to painful stimulation.

A key finding was that people who live with chronic pain have higher levels of cortisol than healthy people. Also, those with a smaller hippocampus tend to have more cortisol, and are likely to feel more pain. They have a stronger response to stress, which makes pain worse, and which then makes chronic pain more debilitating over time. So, basically, people with a smaller hippocampus, and those who feel the effects of stress worse than others, face a higher risk of long-lasting pain. That's why managing stress is vital.

There are many ways to manage stress in your life, and it may be helpful to begin with a visit to a psychologist, reiki practitioner, or yoga teacher, all of whom can provide very insightful tips. There are also some easy remedies you can start doing today, like exercising regularly and joining a yoga, pilates, or tai chi class. Meditation and aromatherapy are also good ways of keeping your stress levels low. When you feel bogged down by stress, it's easy to think that it will never go away, but several tools are mentioned in this book that can help ease your stress fears. Take the fitness chapter, with its yoga and exercise workouts, or the meditation section in this chapter, not to mention the wonderful foods we can eat to help us feel healthy and relaxed.

Here are some gems to help you stop stress:

- Switch off the 'lizard voice' from your ancient brain by creating change. Different destinations and new friendships will keep the human brain evolving.
- Don't veg out in front of boring TV; get on the internet or read a book and learn new ideas.
- Make the effort to do things you love.
- Use shamanic day dreaming to see your future.
- Still the monkey brain by becoming the watcher within, through meditation.
- Do creative things in your life; this expression calms stressful thoughts.
- Seek out spiritual or inspirational workshops and hobbies to self-discover and evolve who you are – your true self. This will stop your frontal lobes shrivelling up into boredom.

Remember that meditation teaches you to evolve your mind. It takes you away from fear and reactive responses to life and allows you to become a witness, have a restful awareness, give intuitive responses and ask why things should happen. It then takes you to a creative intuitive response and a visionary manifesting state of mind, and finally to a sacred source of intelligence that moves beyond a rational mind and taps into a cosmic intelligence.

The elders say that when we ask about life and we knock on the door, when the door finally opens, it opens from the inside. If you avoid toxic places and relationships, and if you heal and love each other, the world and the universe will reward you with a longer, healthier life. It is actually within your power to change your age biologically by up to fifteen years, and this is truly incredible.

Breathing

Another way to live a life with less stress is by being a master of breathing exercises, as breath has been called a natural tranquiliser. According to Andrew Weil, focused intentional breathing makes changes in the body. Weil gives one example, which is called the 4-7-8 breath. What you need to do is place the tip of your tongue on the roof of your mouth, then inhale through the nose for four seconds, hold for seven seconds, and then exhale noisily through the mouth for eight seconds.

NLP

Here I'm going to talk a little about NLP (Neuro-Linguistic Programming). NLP gives us learning tools to change how we feel about things that have happened to us, and there is a key difference to using this technique instead of traditional counselling. With NLP, you do not need to keep replaying memories and changing them. As lawyers demonstrate in court with leading questions, memories are not hardwired, and you stand a chance of reinforcing the condition by repeatedly revisiting the problems of the past. Switching phobias off and on, as well as traumatic memories, is a highly evolved skill, but it can be achieved by using NLP.

I remember when I was on a head trauma ward and I was told to tilt table (where the patient is effectively standing up, strapped to the table) a man who'd had his frontal lobes removed; the surgeon said he had simply cut out the problem! For me it felt like I was working with a pile of clothes, not a human being. I've also been on high security psychiatric units with inmates drugged up to the hilt, where a similar attitude was used. It shouldn't be this way.

I was fortunate enough to get my NLP certification under Richard Bandler – one of the co-creators of this methodology, along with John Grinder – and personally, I have found my basic knowledge useful in uncovering multiple personalities, especially those created through trauma, where the patient's memory is associated with that specific trauma. We can easily have two or three different personalities, all at different times and with subtle differences in our tone, speed of speaking and our pain levels. There will be more of this in my next book, *The Human Garage*.

Anyway, we all learn in a variety of ways, including visual, auditory, and kinaesthetic methods, and on stage I have learnt a lot about communicating my views in different ways so that everyone in the audience understands it. For example, I used puppets and colourful items for visual-oriented people, and movement on stage for kinaesthetically wired souls. Again, there will be more in *The Human Garage* as this is a treatment tool as well.

Hypnosis

Whenever I say hypnosis to my patients, you can see them looking for the pocket watch and an eerie voice commanding immoral zombie-like actions while they reply, "Yes, Master." Sadly, that isn't the case – it's not that exciting. The truth is that the patient remains hypervigilant and in control at all times, with complete free will.

I am trained in this, though I rarely use it unless I know my client well. On top of this, I have witnessed fascinating past life regression work and have also been a subject myself on occasion. If you are interested in having this done or learning about it, just make sure that the person is well qualified and you will be safe.

F.E.T

Just a quick mention here, as this psychological acupressure is helpful when you are anxious or when you are needing a tool to cope with painful memories, and it is said to work by releasing blockages in the energy system that are of an emotional intensity. These blockages lead to limiting beliefs, adding to addictive, compulsive, anxious, and depressive behaviours. More and more medics are using these techniques to help with chronic pain and illness.

Basically, you tap on a recipe of acupressure points in sequence: side of hand, inner eyebrow, outer under eye, above lip, medial end collar bones, and under the armpits. While doing so, you say a mantra, such as, "Even though I have (insert problem or issue here), I truly, deeply love myself." You don't tap any rude bits, by the way!

I came across these techniques years ago with some American and Canadian clients who explained to me that the methods date back to ancient acupuncture days, thousands of years ago. My information is from American colleagues, however, if you do an internet search there are lots of free resources available in the UK as well. Gary Craig's website – www.emofree.com – for instance, offers a wealth of information as well as free downloads, which you can use as a self-help tool.

Let's Meditate On Life

Personally, I have always found meditation useful when reducing stress and anxiety. Beyond this, it has a higher purpose: to rediscover our true nature. When our minds are uncluttered we make better choices, and therefore we become happier and healthier. When we learn to look deeper into the way we think about the world – and especially our purpose for being here, and the way we communicate this – our whole way of living can radically change. This is when relationships blossom.

There is evidence to suggest that the human brain is still evolving, and the proof of its historical development is housed within the brain architecture itself. Modern day MRI (Magnetic Resonance Imaging) has allowed us to start understanding the way we use our minds. Something I find fascinating is that ancient knowledge actually supports these modern day scientific findings, with the only real difference being the language and symbols used to describe it.

In ancient cultures, people were very much part of nature; they treated the earth with reverence and worship, and believed that their healthy existence depended on having this outlook. Shamans – who pre-date our modern day doctors – were masters of meditation and medicine. Unfortunately, these ancient healers, these guardians of the Earth, were forced into secrecy by so-called religious invaders, who stole their lands and tortured those who spoke of the old ways.

The Four Levels of Perception

Let me briefly share with you how you can look at problems in a fresh way by using ancient knowledge. During my research and my travels, I have come across many shamanic teachings that describe the four levels of perception. These are the serpent, the jaguar, the hummingbird, and the eagle, and as you read on, you may recognise your own predominant way of thinking in one of these.

The serpent represents the part of the brain that we share with lizards and reptiles, and we need this in order to work well in crisis situations; it is about survival and instinctive needs, and it holds a very material perception. Dominant lizard-brained people take care of business in a very practical way, but they are not always too pleasant to be around.

The jaguar perception is all to do with the mammalian brain, called the amygdala or limbic system. This way of looking at the world is built on the reptilian perception, but has added curiosity, care, compassion, sharing, social interaction, and loving. With our belief system, we see what we believe to be true and we share this way with all mammals. In this state of mind, we can break free of old habits with just one single new insight.

The hummingbird is the 'soul of the brain', and it encases the other two and embraces such experiences as imagery, music, poetry, and dreaming. This is housed in the neocortex, which evolved 100,000 years ago, and here we look with reason, visualising and creating solutions within a world seen full of meaning. We also embrace wellbeing.

Finally, the eagle perception is housed in the prefrontal cortex, which is known as the 'God' brain, and it has been described as, "God experiencing itself through man". Here we look with concerns about the planet, quantum mechanics, the future, pollution, and big picture solutions to big problems.

Meditation is the doorway to explore how you think about problems such as these. Where do you predominantly operate from?

Meditating On Chakras

This ancient knowledge is 1000 years old, and can be found in both Chinese and Tibetan history. Its focus is on chi, the seed of your genius, and they say that if you can harness your chi, your serpent power spreads throughout your body like Niagara Falls, rather than just a stream, which is what so many of us experience.

Kundalini is the name given to the serpent energy that rests coiled in your base chakra, and it represents the union between Shakti and Shakta. It is said to have its own sense of purpose to enlightenment, with great paranormal gifts and great spiritual purpose and awareness. Through meditation, this divine spark travels up through energetic currents in your spine, combining with universal energy and then showering and cleansing the body, burning up old karma. It is believed to be our primary force within us, and is often painted in red and orange colours.

There are Kundalini exercises within reiki training – however, if you are interested, find a tutor, as for the un-initiated, these exercises are a little racy for my book. I will instead take you through a brief, gentle meditative relaxation exercise to enhance the spiritual wellbeing of your chakras.

Firstly, let us briefly understand the essence of our chakra personalities. Our chakras – those spinning vortices of energy, of which there are seven major ones along the spine, 21 minor and 700 mini chakras (acupuncture points) – each have their own functions for maintaining health. The seven main ones are part of this complex system of energy and expression of consciousness. There are said to be 72,000 nadis in the body, which are small, fine energy communication channels between the chakras and the meridian lines. Three of these channels run along the spine, and the central one is talked about in yoga where 'the winds' and elements lead to enlightenment. This is described as a silver cord with a red middle, the channel on the left being lunar energy, with purifying and nourishing being on the right solar.

The fundamental life force of the person resides in the base chakra, which is the one called Kundalini, and as the body is cleansed through the chakras and nadis, consciousness and a powerful awakened state develops to achieve all life's goals and to fulfil life's purpose. It is said in ancient texts that outside the body resides the aura, which is comprised of seven subtle bodies making up the energy field that emanates from the human body: physical, etheric, emotional, mental, intuitive, monadic, and the divine. My healer friends can often either feel or see them. The etheric receives and transmits vital energy from the chakras, which then goes on to connect with emotional energies, then thoughts, then the divine. This is a huge subject and not one for this book, but those of you who go on to study meditation, yoga and chi kung will come across this.

Briefly, here are the seven chakras, as they are discussed in Western interpretations of reiki, crystal healing, meditation and yoga. Here are a few key words associated with each to consider in chakra meditations:

- **Root Chakra:** foundation of energy, survival, colour red, fear and anger, assertiveness, physical attraction, desire to create new inventions, to do, move, express, act, to know how, confidence, individual integrity, its purpose to become solid ground or no value in placing a spiritual ladder onto it, it is an anchor to spiritual balanced energy.

- **Sacral Chakra:** pain is held here, emotional shock is held here, colour is orange.
- **Solar Plexus Chakra:** know thyself, self-identity, personal belief systems, the organiser, librarian of experiences, comfort or fear, colour yellow.
- **Heart Chakra:** how we reach out and touch other people, love, balance, acceptance, relationships, beliefs, pink with green hues.
- **Throat Chakra:** finding your voice, communication, language, sound, speaking our truth unblocked by others' values and beliefs and our life's trauma. Blue is the associated colour.
- **Third Eye Chakra:** seeing the picture, visions, creative dreaming, perception and command, hearing and seeing, consciousness of self, unique personality of mind, we are in our heads and yet can use intuition to see beyond and gain clairvoyant insight. Colour is indigo.
- **Crown Chakra:** main coordinating centre of body, over sits master gland in the brain. It represents illumination, the fountain head, non-emotional, detached from people and objects, the colour violet.

For a month, do a daily short meditation. Start with each chakra – for example, the base – and focus on its meaning and colour as well as its location. Bring awareness to that point for three minutes, focus your attention, and breathe deeply and slowly, breathing through that chakra. When you are happy with that, start again at the base and picture a coiled serpent of fluid energy, as well as a silver cord with a red core through your spine, and expand your Kundalini up through that channel. You may choose to stop and focus on every chakra, or you may want to focus purely on the silver cord, and like mercury in a thermometer, let the energy rise.

This is just a brief example of how an early culture used the power of the mind. Many cultures and philosophies – including that of Buddhism – meditate, and some of the most successful people on the planet have learnt the ancient secrets to mastering the power of the mind. Learning to move through different levels of perception brings awareness and the opportunity to live an enriched and happy life.

By harnessing the power of the mind, we can open ourselves up to all kinds of alternative thinking and beliefs that will not only benefit us, but which can benefit others as well. By learning all of these different techniques, we can help friends and relatives who are ill, making a real difference in their lives while they're still here. There is so much we can do to comfort them and make their lives less painful, and you'll be able to learn more about this in the lifestyle chapter.

I'll leave you with this quote by US philosopher, psychologist, and physician, William James, as you consider this chapter and how changing your own mindset can change the way you live your life.

"Human beings, by changing the inner attitudes of their minds, can change the outer aspects of their lives." (William James, 1842 – 1910).

Now, let's look at some more real life case studies that really exemplify the importance of being in the right mindset. All names have been changed to protect the identities of all involved.

An Example of What the Power of Belief Can Achieve

Having attended a couple of Tony Robbins UPW (Unleash the Power Within) firewalks, I was fascinated to think about what made thousands of people – both in Rome and London – happily walk over glowing coals, without burning their feet. It seemed to be some kind of cleverly orchestrated crowd excitement, tipping the people into a trancelike euphoric state. On both occasions, I watched in awe at the sheer enthusiasm of people who were doing something that the intelligent part of the brain should be rejecting, and quite frankly, at which it should be screaming, "No!"

Joseph McClendon and Tony Robbins can whip a crowd into a frenzy strong enough to jump off a cliff, should they suggest they could, and this fascinated me enough to present with Joseph in Europe. The idea of walking over hot coals originated in Brazil in the 6th Century, when monks believed that this walk purified and healed. They said acupuncture points burned at the point where the illness was, and every year, the Kannon Buddhists still do this on Buddha's birthday. It just goes to show the power of belief and what it can do for us. Here are some more stories about what our minds are capable of.

Enthused by Tony and Joseph's UPW effect on people's mindsets, I happily agreed to write and present on pain at the Z factor for a couple of summer seminars in Southern Spain. Last time, I took puppets to engage with the audience and to tell true stories of patient tales, each one designed to ignite a, 'that's me!' moment. I am careful to use composite stories, meaning that I mix together their profession, gender, objective and subjective history – like a cut and paste – to protect the patients; even though I have their permission, I don't want any strangers knowing their story unless told by themselves in person or video. It was a privilege to be part of a life changing event where people actually started to understand that the environment has a big impact on your health and happiness. It was so empowering.

Spanish Wedding

A lovely couple who lived up in the hills, not far from where we were presenting, came to talk to me. There was an important wedding coming up and the woman had a broken bone. Casts and dresses don't look great on camera, so they took a trip to my UK practice, and we accelerated the bone repair with MRT. With this – and with her mindset being so strong – she needed no plaster just three weeks after the break, which was great for her, but which confused the hell out of her Spanish doctor! Her state of mind really helped her body to heal, which is something I see time and time again and cannot stress enough.

Mind Over Matter –
A Painful Memory Left a Deep Imprint

Earlier this year, a gentle soul came to see me. Retired head teacher Alice had limped badly for fifty years, believing that she had to move that way because her spine was twisted, and because her leg was too short on one side. A rather large lady, she came into my clinic – clutching her MRI scan like a death sentence – and explained to me that she believed this was her lot in life. She had many coloured pills, and her GP had told her that there was nothing else to be done. Her spinal MRI showed disc degeneration with facet joint arthritis. It wasn't excessive for her age, but it was enough to give her pain.

Although her husband had died a few years ago, she had a lot of friends, including her favourite horse. She actually had a stable full of horses, but with one in particular, they'd been inseparable for over ten years. Her lifestyle and diet were green, although pain had taken its toll, and depression had reduced her desire to exercise, so her mind and fitness were red.

I could tell by listening to her that there was something else; something deep inside her that was partly accountable for her pain. There were thoughts that were firing up her mindset and emotions, and chiselling her patterns of movement. There was a deep sadness inside her.

There was also a lot of compensatory posture with her, and I found out that her favourite horse also limped; his arthritis was raging, and it wasn't helped by the rider's posture, as Alice rode him in a strange way. This, therefore, became a fixed problem for both horse and rider. Arthritis loves stiff joints, and so it moved in.

So, how did I treat Alice? Step One was to give her some weaning insoles. These gently teased her away from the manner in which she believed she had to move, and also adjusted the leg length and corrected the pelvic torsion. I asked her to ride her horse again and see what happened, as we needed to take it slow for his sake too.

Step Two was to teach her some home exercises and stretches, as her body was changing throughout the treatment programme. We also increased hydration levels and Quad scanned her, which is a specialist technology that looks at cellular health.

Step Three was to give her MRT (Magnetic Resonance Treatment), to help repair the damaged cartilage tissue within the discs and facet joints. I then assessed this wonderful lady's back, to seek out both her neuropathic pain and her beliefs about her pain; as limbs are an extension of the spine, her limp would be associated with this.

I am well known for releasing nerve tissue deep in the back, with the patient awake, and by using a laser and a dry needle articulated in a plunger (ouch). Deep muscle contractures can be evidence of an old injury and are laden with emotional memories. When an emotional trigger is fired, a huge white cell memory immune response occurs. This initially gives a massive healing reaction of more pain as the pain factor increases and the inflammation surges.

We talked while I used gentle reiki techniques, and I also dry needled some more deep contractures in her spine. She told me she felt the same deep ache as when she'd felt her back tear while giving birth to her children all those years ago. You see, Alice had become pregnant with twins as a teenager, and with no financial support, she was forced to give up the babies and have them adopted. She had kept her pain through all those years; she'd actually anchored her childbirth trauma pain in her back. This realisation was a big physical and emotional release that she could now walk away from.

Unfortunately, the next day the vet had to put her favourite horse to sleep, as his arthritis was beyond help, and they had to end his suffering. MRT is still in the research stage for horses. We wept together.

The good news is that she felt so physically and mentally strong from her treatment that she could handle it. She even took on a new job looking after the horses on a kid's farm at a local stately home. I gently reminded her that this shouldn't be possible – after all, wasn't she supposed to be disabled and in pain?!

So, what does this story tell us? Physical pain, a loss of confidence, and depression can all result from a locked-in emotional pain. When something is too great to bear emotionally, the subconscious employs a defence mechanism, dumping it into a physical manifestation that we then don't know how to deal with. By following the pain back to its very real but invisible cause, I could treat Alice using the correct knowledge – something which her GP didn't have the time or the resources to find out about. Mindset is a very powerful thing.

You Can't Cut Away Pain
Where There Isn't Any

One day, this rather rotund gentle soul came trundling up the creaky stairs in my clinic, with her very caring partner in tow. Her name was Eileen, and she was a lollipop lady, so walking across roads was actually in her job description. She seemed in a bad way, and there was pain written all over her face. Her traffic light scores on the doors were: fitness – red. Lifestyle – green. Mindset – red. Diet – red. She limped badly and was bent forward, clearly in a lot of pain.

"It's my foot!" she told me, looking down at her large boot. "I can't sleep, I can't drive, I can't walk, I can't even think straight. I can't help with the gardening or the housework, anything. I'm so depressed, I just want to chop it off. Help me!"

Giving her a sympathetic ear, I asked her to tell me her story.

"I've been in pain every second of every day for six months," she said. "I had a very painful foot, especially on the bottom part, so they cut a tight muscle underneath, the one called the plantar fascia. It felt even sorer after so they put me in a pot, and when it came out, it was even worse. This is why I've got this big boot, as well as having lots of injections and lots of pills. It's even sorer now. They wanted to block my nerves, but I got too scared. Then I found you."

I wanted to find out why Eileen wasn't healing. Her optimum health wasn't good, and she had become – understandably – very upset. She wasn't exercising at all, and she had a lot of extra adipose tissue due to consuming too many calories. I asked her if she liked walking and exercising, and her partner raised his eyebrows. I took that as a no. The foot pain was creating a behavioural pattern of belief that it was reasonable for her to stop moving and eat everything in sight in order to comfort herself.

She was in such pain, and she just kept saying she wanted her foot cutting off; she just couldn't wait to be rid of this agony. Instead, I asked if I could assess her, and on closer examination, it became apparent that her lumbar back was weak, and that it was being made worse by a lack of exercise and by her weight.

For Step One, I gently spoke to her about her belief regarding her pain. This meant carefully broaching the subject that her problem was actually in the nerve root, coming through a little tunnel at the side of the lumbar spine. I talked to her about an integrated medical approach, and about how wonderful it was that her surgeon was open enough to send her to see me. In the UK, neurology is separate to orthopaedics, with all specialists working in isolation. The trouble is, the body doesn't know this.

I had to stop her fixation on cutting off her foot, instead directing her attention to curing the origin of her back pain. Without criticising any other colleagues, I gently explained to her where the problem was, and then I conducted IMS (Intramuscular Stimulation) on her, using Professor Gunn's method. This is an ingenious treatment for chronic pain, involving a laser, dry needling, and cutting through muscle contractures. This then releases any trapped nerves.

Fifteen minutes after she left my clinic, all the pain melted away. Her beliefs had been smashed. Here was a lady, prepared – and actually wanting – to have her foot cut off, and the pain was gone after just one session. Now she could install new beliefs regarding her body and her health, which will help the next time she has an issue like this.

Step Two was to get her to sustain her health. I pointed out two key areas that she could improve on – the food she was eating and the exercise she should be doing – and gave her positive mantras for her to be able to do this (as she had told me that she comfort eats and hates exercise of any kind).

The real hero of this story was her surgeon, who embraced the neuropathic tale of pain. The message in this story is that limbs are an extension of the spine, and that you often need to look there to see what the real problem is. Never let this lady's experience happen to you; look after your spine.

It is incredible to think that Eileen was willing to actually have her foot cut off, when all she needed was a bit of treatment and to change the way she thought about her injury. In order to save her foot, we had to change her belief system – another illustration of the power of the mind.

This story reminds me of a trip I took to Malta. After having a podiatric surgeon at my practice for a couple of years, he taught me about painkilling injections and I taught him about how faulty nerves in the lower back can be the cause of foot pain. As a result of this, I found myself on a little plane off to Malta to present our work to the podiatrist's convention. Well, I had a great time! It must be the sun and living on a small rock, but it was a lot of fun sharing my knowledge, and I have great memories of friendly drivers and amazingly long dinners.
What struck me most was that they found stripping naked – apart from pants, of course; please, we're British! – as terrifying as they did feet, and I tried to put

their minds at rest. I explained that I was more discreet than my professor, and told them a true, humorous story about him to illustrate this fact. While teaching on stage at Cambridge University, he actually popped out another professor's testicles to demonstrate S1 nerve impact on them, and this was in front of his step mother – a young Chinese lady – who promptly fainted! This, however, did not make my current crowd feel any better, so we compromised with the clothing.

The moral of Eileen's story is that the cause of pain – in this case, foot pain – can be coming from somewhere else.

——◦○◦——

Nothing to Fear but Fear Itself

One day, a man named William came into my clinic. He was eighty years old, he was a softly spoken chap, and he was walking with a cane and had a caring wife hanging off his arm. He'd recently been in hospital after falling in his green house and now he felt that his leg was weak. He was told that he'd suffered a stroke and that the only way he was going to get better was to take a lot of pills and get a lot of rest. His diagnosis, however, was uncertain, as both a brain scan and ECG were all clear.

I asked him for his story, and he told me that he had been caring for his granddaughter (including lifting her) before his stroke. Now he wouldn't lift her, and he also wasn't swimming as much as he used to. His memory was a little poorer now and he was scared to go out in case he had another stroke. His wife, however, was insistent – she had done Girl Guide first aid and was convinced that he hadn't had a stroke at all.

So, no lifting, less exercise... guess what I was thinking? I did the traffic light health check, and while his diet and lifestyle were green (he had good family support), his exercise and his mindset were both red. He was terrified. Every time he tried to do something vaguely physical, his mind would shout at him: "You've had a stroke! Stop what you're doing! You might die!"

The hero in this story is his wife, with her unbending faith that he would get through this. She understood that his mindset wasn't strong enough to sustain his life, unless she could help to clear his thoughts. She realised that she couldn't stay angry with him, and she also knew that she had to hold his hand throughout the process. She believed she could transform both her fear and his.

So, back at my clinic, I looked at all of the evidence and traced his symptoms back to a section in the mid-lumbar spine, where one vertebra was slightly raised out over the next.

For Step One, I placed a needle in a tight contracture about the guilty nerve root, causing him to scream. Once my ears had stopped ringing, I thought, 'Gotcha!' I told him that his wife was right, and that he may not have had a stroke; the specific reflex change and the muscle weakness and numbness built good evidence for a case against a stroke, instead pointing to spinal stenosis, which is very common in the elderly. In terms of back pain, it is usually one of the following: mechanical, poor posture, or lack of exercise, a trapped nerve, disc, or stenosis, or a more serious pathology. I ruled out the latter explanation by asking his doctor to do all of the normal blood tests.

Step Two was to rebuild his confidence. I told him that I'd write to his medic and clear my diagnosis, and then I told him that we'd get him swimming. I also told him he could take the cane he'd been using to walk with and use it for his tomato plants instead. Due to his poor memory, I made sure to repeat this comforting information to him. I also asked his wife to do reiki on him at home, which she did while playing soft music and repeating soft words to settle his mind.

Step Three was to rebuild his spinal muscles, and I gave him a programme of exercises that he could do at home.

Step Four was to change his belief that he was dying – which is what he honestly thought was happening. We had to convince him he wasn't, and make him change his mindset accordingly.

Was there a happy ending? Yes there was. After his IMS treatment, he got up, shocked and surprised. He said that he felt different and could walk much more easily. A later MRI scan confirmed stenosis, which had been made worse by the fall. There was no spinal tumour, and he hadn't had a stroke. He was a lucky man, with a loving, caring wife.

He had nothing to fear but fear itself, if only he could remember what he was so fearful about! The message here is that it can still take a lot of convincing once a belief is formed, even when all of the physical symptoms have gone. Reinforcement is paramount.

Head and Heart and Never the Twain Shall Meet

Another time, a tall, dignified gentleman strode into my clinic office in a very dapper suit, clutching a bible. In a clear, posh voice, he said, "It's my neck, it's a pain. I've had marvellous surgery and it's bolted back together, but the damn thing keeps giving me pain."

This man was called Brian, and he liked to look after himself – his diet and exercise levels were good. However, I detected a problem in his mindset and his lifestyle (where his diet and exercise results were green, his mindset and lifestyle results were amber).

He had a strong religious calling and faith. His neck showed signs of wear beyond the surgery, and his overall movement was reasonable. When he took his tie off and lay down, however, everything changed. As I placed my hands on his throat, I intuitively felt a chill, a deep sense of loss, and a lack of ability to communicate his feelings about it. I sensed a tightening, an evil end to a close one's life, and Brian's inability to let go of that person.

Through sobs, I gently probed his neck while he told me about the murder of his daughter. He spoke with angry, desperate words. Then, it all made sense. There was a huge heart and head disconnect – the battle with his faith and what had happened to his child. His need to process this emotional pain had manifested itself as a somatic pain in his neck.

His orthodox surgeon believed that he had cut out his pain, but he hadn't, as you can't simply 'cut out' an emotional pain this deep. Brian's neck pain gave him an excuse to talk to someone and to not appear weak to his peers, who believed that praying to God should give him all the comfort he needed. He was not, as yet, ready to let go of his daughter, and he had to have a vehicle through which to express his emotions.

I needed to quieten any physical pain without awakening the deeper giant within – at least, not until he was ready to go on this journey with me. As it was, he was emotionally gagged. His tie was his disconnect – his brain wasn't permitted to process the painful heart and therefore, when he wore his tie, the two were separated. Make no mistake: strong, emotional damage can present itself as a physical pain for life, if not helped.

Instinctively, I wanted to rescue him. It was his soul that was in more torment than his arthritic neck, and the transition had to be gentle. As someone who practises integrative medicine, knowing when to step back is very important. The lesson here is the importance of symbolism. As soon as Brian took off his tie, I could sense what was really bothering him, and it wasn't just the pain in his neck. The message of a business suit and tie is that, 'You will hear from my head, not my heart'. A loosening of the tie means, 'I will open up more to you'. After all, how many men make love with their tie on?!

Brian is still on his pain-relief journey, as he's slowly coming to terms with what happened, and what he needs to do in order to be free of his pain.

When Ignorance Really Is Bliss

While this story has a sad ending, it is illustrative of how the mind can either help or hinder your healing.

A lovely lady by the name of Fiona came to see me with her best friend, Wendy, who was around fifty years old and had a back ache complaint. Before I met Wendy, however, Fiona informed me that her friend had a huge cancerous tumour on her back, which had curved her spine. Wendy wasn't aware that it was cancerous, as she had asked not to know her diagnosis, so I treated her using a mixture of reiki and gentle acupuncture to ease her pain.

Fiona and Wendy's husband were both aware that Wendy was on borrowed time, and that the tumour was just too large – she'd soon die. As per her request, however, they didn't tell Wendy. You see, Wendy wanted to be around to see her daughter get married, and she did. Then she wanted to be around to see her granddaughter, which she also did. Even though the doctors had given Wendy just a few short months to live, she lived for five more years, as she didn't know the truth about her condition.

One day, however, it became clear to her husband that it was too serious not to keep his wife informed, and so he told her that she had cancer, but that it was treatable (which it wasn't). Wendy went through chemotherapy and radiotherapy, and survived. Although her spine was still in a horrible shape, the pain wasn't too bad. The doctors couldn't believe she was still alive – surely, it was impossible?

Feeling guilty about not telling Wendy the truth, her husband took her to the hospital and told her everything. They showed her the scan and told her that it wasn't, in fact, treatable at all. After years of living, she died within three days.

Not a very happy ending, I'm sure you'll agree, but it really does tell us a lot about our mindset and how our minds can affect what happens to our bodies. It is an incredibly powerful thing.

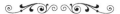

Once you've read this chapter, please go to page 247 of the appendix and complete the traffic light questionnaire for mindset again to see how you have improved.

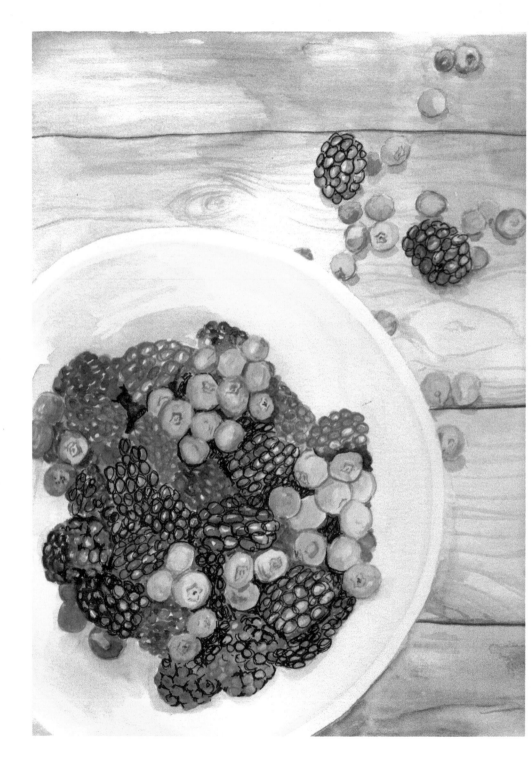

Nutrition And Hydration

Let Your Spirit Shine Through!

You have an inner jewel. Let your spirit, the divine gem, shine through, and create a radiance about you wherever you go.

Let your mind be planted with seeds of love and joy and hope, and courage and universal goodwill and opulent harvest shall grow.

Think of each year as a sower scattering these seeds in your heart; then water them with the dews of sympathy, and throw open the windows to the broad sunlight of heaven while they ripen.

And – as surely as the days
come and go –
so surely
shall your
life grow.

– *Ella Wheeler Wilcox*

Before you read this chapter, please go to page 248 of the appendix and complete the traffic light questionnaire for nutrition and hydration.

⁘

I am sure you have heard about lemmings, those little animals that supposedly follow their leader and all jump off a cliff to their deaths. Now, if we look at human behaviour, much of what we do is very lemming-like. For example, just look at fashion. Some remote group decides what the 'in look' and colour is going to be for next year, then promote it like mad, and everyone buys it to be 'in fashion'. It doesn't matter how bad or uncomfortable some of the fashion is; we follow it to fit in. Don't be a lemming this January and follow some fad diet! Instead, give your body all the nutrients it needs, and exercise wisely.

Now, some of you are probably thinking, 'I wouldn't do that, I've got too much common sense', but have you ever thought about what 'common sense' actually means? Something can only be sensible if it's already known to us. Fire is dangerous, don't play with it: that's common sense, right? No, not necessarily. It is only common sense if we have previously experienced what fire does. A couple of years ago I was watching a programme about polar bears, and one bear came close to this Canadian village, the residents of which were burning their rubbish in a sizeable bonfire. The bear clearly had no idea what fire was and just walked up to it and stuck a paw in, only to run off yelping. That bear was probably unique after that incident, in being the only polar bear to have the sense to know that fire is dangerous.

Using Food as Medicine to Stay Out of Pain

We all overindulge in the winter, especially with the run up to Christmas, and this is the time when we all suffer from the most colds. Actually, in the months of February, March and April, we have more colds and achy joints than ever in the UK, as our immune system is suffering from our rich diet, as well as our lack of raw fresh fruit, vegetables, and sunshine.

The problem here lies in the fact that for the majority of us, the health risks associated with a very rich and acid diet are not known and are therefore no more 'common sense' than fire was to the polar bear. However, at least the bear learnt very quickly that fire was dangerous and would be very wary the next time he came across it. The implications of poor diet – and more importantly, a far too acidic diet – are not immediately apparent. Even worse, the fact that 'everybody else' in an individual's social group is doing the same thing, means that it doesn't even register that a diet may be poor in the first place.

No better example of this can be given than a highly publicised TV programme shown a few years ago, which monitored the health implications of junk food by getting a volunteer to live on nothing other than junk. He actually had to be taken off the diet because his health plummeted so rapidly. What impact has this had? Very little, if you look at the explosion of junk food outlets. So, this January don't waste money on fad diets, just do a little reading about healthy food, drink more water, and use natural pain killing foods with natural anti-inflammatories.

The Wrong Food Feeds Pain

Most of us eat too much of the food that enhances pain, and too little of the food that reduces pain. Soil nutrients are not what they used to be, as they have more additives, more are being processed, and more have a longer shelf life. Our cells depend on food and water for creating healing, energy and cleansing, but because of the poor food we eat (which has additives and is heavily processed), we have persistent inflammation contributing to musculoskeletal pain, arthritis, diabetes, heart attacks, strokes, cancer... you name it. Refined grains, omega 6 fats, too much sugar, and too much dairy – especially milk – all stress the system out, and pain due to too much inflammation damages nerves beyond any injury, and also causes tissue pain in the tendons, ligaments, and joints.

Our ancestors were hunters and gatherers who lived on a planet with a relatively low population, where the soil was rich in nutrients with hardly any toxic chemicals. They ate fresh meat, berries, roots (therefore, a lot of healthy omega 3 oils), and fruit and vegetables high in antioxidants. They had no processed foods, no wheat, no trans fats, no excess sugar or omega 6 and no processed dairy. Even if you eat some of these foods yourself, pulling some fresh vegetables out of your garden – from well fertilised soil – is a small start. For our ancestors, their healthy diet helped to control chronic inflammation, something which pervades the modern day Western lifestyle.

We are becoming increasingly obese, including our children. We are a fat nation, and because of this, we find ourselves in a major health crisis. This extra fat not only strains our joints, but these engorged fat cells fire off inflammation. Organ fat is crawling with immune cells, prolonging inflammation and damaging the surrounding tissue. Living longer means that these days, a lot more of us are over 35, and around this age, our natural pain blocking anti-inflammatories (proteolytic enzymes) dry up. We are, essentially, rotting, as these are the guys that usually help to shut the pain gate in the dorsal horn of the spinal cord. Our next generation is not going to live longer than us, and this is the first time in history that this has happened – it says a lot, doesn't it? Due to needing more help in order to control our body and not getting it, we make too much fibrin, causing too much scar tissue in our tendons, skin, and joints. This then causes arthritis, fibromyalgia, artery narrowing, and poor healing all round. I now have ground breaking technology at my practice that puts the clock back on joints, however, cells still need a healthy environment in which to flourish in the first place.

The Okinawa Project

I have always held a quiet fascination for the Okinawa project (Willcox, Willcox and Suzuki, 1996). There is a question (a favourite of the much admired Bruce Lipton) that is often asked by people in my profession: how much is health due to our genes and how much is due to the environment? Just after I started my intense pain studying – which took me off to both Canada and Korea – a group of doctors and scientists asked that Holy Grail question about longevity and took off to the Japanese island of Okinawa to find the answer. This group of Canadian medical research scientists were led by Dr Suzuki, and they succeeded in unlocking the keys to biological and psychospiritual behaviours in healthy people who had young arteries, little heart disease, healthy breast and prostrates, strong bones, sharp and happy minds, and slim bodies.

They discovered that lifelong exercise (tai chi and aerobic exercise) was vital to both toning their bodies and reinforcing their belief systems towards longevity. They had nutrient and mineral-rich water, and a healing, mostly plant-based died that included soy, fish, veggies, and the right kinds of fats. They had a strong social and community spirit with a self-responsibility attitude to health, a profound reverence for nature, and a deep respect for each other, using a blend of Taoism and Confucianism. Women are the spiritual keepers of the bonds between old and new society, and the elders are revered. Their philosophy – and their obligation – is to help whenever a fellow human fails.

Here are the scores on the doors for these guys: mindset – green. Food and water – green. Fitness – green. Lifestyle – green. Get my point? These 181 pretty, palm-laden islands hold a key to longevity. The four main killers in our Western world – cancer, heart disease, stroke, and reactions to drugs – do not darken their shores. If the USA shared their health levels, at least 80% of coronary care units would close and 33% of cancer wards. This island, which drinks in the China Sea, is the land of immortals.

The Okinawa way echoes a lot of what my book is about; their diet alone is a powerful way of ageing slowly and decreasing suffering, which they wrap up in good old-fashioned values, morals and beliefs. At that time, there was a flood of scientific papers which supported the notion that what we do affects our health and longevity, and back in the late 90s – when this project was being discovered – there were early stirrings to believing at least 2/3 of gene expression was in part due to the food we eat, and the rest due to lifestyle, exercise and mindset: the four keys, in effect.

Three migration studies featuring diet and heart disease (the Ni-hon-san study featuring Japanese living in Japan, Honolulu and San Francisco, the Honolulu Heart Program, and migration studies of Okinawans in Okinawa and Brazil) demonstrated that when lifestyle and diet is changed, arteries do not, because we are born with different genes. It is the environmental expression of genes.

Acidosis and Acid Alkaline Diet

The food we consume contains essential nutrients that are needed to maintain normal metabolic function. However, lots of diets fail to include these and so unbalance our body chemistry. Hence, after an indulgent Christmas, the fad diets that always emerge with gusto in January are not always a healthy choice.

Now, this is going to puzzle and surprise you. Many of us have heard about sugar tests, cholesterol, hormones and – some of you – homocysteine. For more information, have a look at *The H Factor* by Dr James Braly and Patrick Holford (Piatkus, 2003), and you can send away for tests from the York lab by looking in the resources section of this book.

Let's return to a simple measurement you can make: how many of you measure your saliva pH as a predictor of health and good diet? Different parts of our body do have slightly different pH levels, but in the main, the absolutely ideal pH falls in a narrow range of mildly alkaline. For more on this, read *The PH Miracle for Weight Loss* by Dr Robert Young and Shelley Young (Grand Central Life & Style, 2006).

I will explain briefly what pH means. The acid/alkaline relationship is quantified on a scale of 1 to 14. Neutral is at 7, above is alkaline, and below is acidic. The body will go into chaos if the correct balance is not achieved; the pH of our bodily fluids critically affects every cell. Chronic over acidity upsets cellular functioning, our thought processes, our breathing, and our heart rate. In fact, here's a little gem for you: if you are slightly fatter, it may be due to being a little acidic. Eating more alkalising food, such as green veggies, will help to slowly rebalance you, as well as drinking more water, which is alkaline. When you are eating better, your skin looks better, and you have more muscle and less fat, as well as having better concentration and physical fitness. You will have fewer energy dips and can benefit from a happier mindset.

Twice Nobel Prize winner Linus Pauling, friend of Einstein and Pat Holford, would always say that nearly all disease can be traced to a mineral deficiency.

Hydration/Water

When we look at hydration, the statistics are staggering: over 80% of the population is dehydrated. In fact, only one person that we've measured at our clinic was actually properly hydrated. For discs in your spine in particular, it is vital that they are properly hydrated, as disc problems can lead to massive pain issues. For good health you need your overall hydration level to be correct, and more specifically, you need the hydration inside and outside your cells to be correct as well. Excess fluid outside the cells is an indication of swelling, and following an operation this can be critical – if too high, this could lead to death.

Within this chapter, I will proceed to explain the body's many calls for water, and the benefits of drinking adequate water are so amazing that it is known as the secret medicine of life. So many of us are wandering around in a constant state of dehydration, with no awareness of this whatsoever. If we don't get enough water, we are walking into a life of chronic painful illness, so you have to think differently about what water is and how much you should put in your body, including how good the water is.

Part of the natural ageing process is that our calls for water are far less obvious, and if we don't do anything about it, there can be dire consequences. It is said that one cup of coffee can take 10 pints of water to rehydrate. One beer 15 pints, and one large soda, 15 litres. However, other research completely denies these diuretic effects, so the jury is still out on that one. What we do know is that all of our bodily functions, all of our cellular activities, depend on hydration.

So, how much should we drink? This is very controversial and an often disputed subject, but generally, these days, people are saying 10 glasses a day, or half your body weight in fluid ounces. Of course, you should check this with your doctor or medical professional to confirm what is right for you personally. Water is necessary for mental agility, the immune system, healing, cleansing, and detoxing, so it is definitely not something that we should ignore.

My favourite water is ionised water (alkaline) – it's delicious. I actually have a Chanson water ioniser at my clinic, thanks to Ronnie Ruiz, our water guru from the Z Factor. Here are a few facts I've gleaned from him over the years that might help you to think differently about the water you're putting in your body.

Ionised water donates electrons to rejuvenate cells, and it mimics free flowing spring water. This water is more 'slippery'; it moves through membranes six times more easily. Negative electrical charge (OH) acts as a powerful antioxidant, absorbing free radicals that can otherwise lead to cell dysfunction. Negative Oxidation Reduction Potential (ORP) produces hydroxyl ions, helps with o2 production, neutralises harmful free radicals, increases energy levels, corrects alkaline/acid balance, hydrates cells, and helps ease stomach acid, as well as reducing ageing properties.

Many chronic degenerative diseases are caused by acidity and dehydration, and if your blood is too acidic, it will rape calcium from bone and magnesium. Acidic waste turns into fatty tissues and then clogs arteries. Furthermore, an acidic, dehydrated environment is associated with crystalline deposits, gout, inflammation and stiffness – water helps to prevent all of this. Microwater is wetter; genetically, the metabolism of our forefathers meant they could absorb water bouncing off natural rock formations, without added chemicals. Make sure you take care when leaving glasses or bottles of water around the place – the water can become more acidic the longer it's left, especially when in a plastic container.

Talking of water, there is a very interesting video on YouTube which shows how the Japanese discovered the health benefits of ionised water back in the 1960s, and since then its use has been medically approved. An ioniser produces both alkaline water, which you drink, and acid water, which you can treat skin conditions with, or if very acidic, you can use to sterilise. The video shows how hospitals are sterilising operating theatres and medical instruments with nothing other than acid water. Surgeons are also shown washing their hands before surgery in nothing other than acid water. This 'miracle' is said to be possible as the water is so acidic that it makes a good cleaning fluid. The irony is that some of the soft drinks we consume are just as acidic as this water. Now you tell me, is it common sense to consume these kinds of drinks? Or is this an example of lemming behaviour?

Poor diet and poor hydration will slowly but surely damage your body and will eventually surface as deteriorating health and disease. You will not get the luxury of an early warning, like the bear did with the fire. Make a decision to commit to a healthier way of living; if you do that, you will live to enjoy many more years to come.

Having said that, being able to measure the health of your cells allows for an early warning of potential problems long before you would normally be aware of them, and we use Quadscan at times to measure both intra and extracellular fluid levels. It is interesting that many patients don't want to know, just in case it's bad news. This is crazy, as its means you are leaving your life to chance, when you could actually plan and control it instead. Expansion of ECW (Extracellular Water) and loss of ICW (Intracellular water) are typical features of systemic illness and this arises from protein leakage into the extra cellular space, as well as the loss of intracellular protein in the case of critical illness. Loss of intracellular potassium and the accumulation of extra cellular sodium result in an increased whole body exchangeable sodium/potassium ratio, which is a strong predictor of mortality in surgical patients.

Being a back specialist, I know that for the health of your spinal discs, it is vital that they are properly hydrated, as disc problems can lead to massive pain problems. As an interesting aside, a doctor known as the 'batman' wrote books about how water helped his fellow inmates in a prison of war camp. His name is Dr Batmanghelidj and he discovered the lifesaving properties of water in the prison of war camp, where prescribing drugs was impossible. His book, *Your Body's Many Cries For Water* (Global Health Solutions, 2008), describes how he believes chronic dehydration damages you, and it is absolutely fascinating.

In December 2003, Dr Batmanghelidj read in the papers about an incredible speech given by a brave chap called Alan (to be discreet), who was then very high up in the GlaxoSmithKline drugs company. He declared that 30 to 50% of the drugs prescribed were known to be ineffective in 90% of the cases, and were still knowingly prescribed by the company. He went on to say that most drugs were ineffective in most cases.

This fuelled the Doc to look into substances with drug-free healing properties. He believed that chronic pain was in part, or at times completely, a signal of chronic dehydration, and so he prescribed 2 1/4 litres of water prior to taking pain killing drugs, due to the dehydrating and toxic effects on cells, especially on the liver. In the prison of war camp, he gave relief to sufferers of peptic ulcers, back pain, and migraine, to name just a few conditions.

His desire to heal in the near impossible conditions of the war camp led to some interesting research, and he became obsessed with the properties of water. Your brain is 85% water, and your body 75% – that makes me feel a very wet creature. When we get a dry mouth, the damage has already been done, as it is a desperate cry for help. As we get older, the signals weaken and the elderly drink less, and if our cells are dehydrated, the mitotic division is not so precise. This is the division of a cell, like a blurred photocopy. You don't want a blurred version of yourself, do you?

There are two life giving properties of water in the body. Firstly, broadly speaking, we have the hydrolytic, a solute composition driving chemical reactions, neurotransmitters, nerve signals, hormones, the continual osmotic flow of substances through a cell membrane, the electrochemical ADP, GTP, and cell battery systems (the cell membrane receptors are the gates to transport in and out of the cell, and they react better in a correctly hydrated environment).

I could relate to Dr. Batmanghelidj's work scientifically within my current work, as hydration levels are important for my MRT clinic to regenerate cartilage. When we suspected patients were not drinking enough, we would Quadscan them. This tells me the hydration levels inside and outside the cells, and directly correlates to the health of that person. If the ratio of water in and outside the cell swings too far, death is unavoidable.

The second life giving property of water is to give structure and shape, like a glue that sticks things together. Water enables an assembly line of packing material to be moved along in a cell to make all the structures needed, including more DNA. I could relate to the importance with my earlier biology research; I had studied histamine release with scanning electron microscopy at different levels of hydration, and the effect was dramatic. At the time, I was looking at the influence of certain cell membrane receptor triggers in asthma, so I understood Dr. Batmanghelidj's work.

This, coupled with Bruce Lipton's lectures and research in the 90s regarding new beliefs about gene expression having a 95% influence on lifestyle, mind, exercise, food and water, and with the big research project in Okinawa, the West started to listen to the possibility of disease being a result – in part – of dehydration.

Food vs. Drugs

Food is better than drugs and it is the key to a healthy future. I find it amazing that currently, only 2% of the world health care fund is spent on preventative health. Our marketing system is aimed at a belief system that equates a long and healthy life with shots, medicines, and diagnostic tests. We know that food can work powerfully in a long-term way that drugs cannot, as it is already a part of our ecosystem; we have evolved to use nutrients that have a system-wide effect throughout our body. Vitamin C and garlic etc. all work synergistically in our complex ecosystem to interact with a complex natural chemistry of food.

Nutritional science has made phenomenal strides and discoveries in recent years. For instance, they know that immunity is strengthened with phytochemicals important to health, and that for a good immune system, you need unrefined plant products. Currently, this makes up only 5% of the American diet (according to the Economics Research Service).

In 2000, a US study showed that a third of deaths were self-inflicted by poor diet, alcohol, smoking, and a lack of exercise (The Journal of the American Medical Association), and epigenetics (the study of environmental factors on genes) has shown that food actually alters the expression of our genes: using food, you can change your genetic predisposition to disease and reprogramme your genes for health (Lichtenstein et al., 2000).

Long-term studies (such as those by the National Intelligence Council) show that the most important factor in preventing chronic disease and premature death is the food we eat (Fuhrman, 2011). Basically, if we don't change our diet, we will eat ourselves to death. In fact, a patient of mine (who is an undertaker) told me that fatter people rot faster, and because of this, they have to be quicker in using the preserving fluid on them compared to slimmer people. Not a nice image, but it makes you think.

Food Switches Genes Off And On

One experiment with mice (poor things) was successful in showing that a change in diet changed their gene expression, and it is a landmark piece of research (Waterland and Jirtle, 2003). They looked at the effects of giving a methyl-rich supplement (folic acid, vitamin B12, betaine, choline) to the mother, who expressed agouti gene fat and had a yellow coat – this predisposes baby mice to cardiovascular problems, diabetes and cancer. Guess what? She gave birth to a healthy, slim, brown mouse, whilst carrying the same genes (Waterland and Jirtle, 2003). Furthermore, Bruce Lipton (who understood how the environment shapes our health) commented on this study, stating how certain methyl proteins can actually silence gene expression (Lipton, 2005). This is because if a methyl group attaches to a gene's DNA, it stops the gene being expressed at all.

Enucleated cells – cells with the DNA removed – can still live on for weeks and respond to stimuli. In fact, cells show intelligent control in the absence of genes, and there will be more on this in my next book. Dr Jeff Bland states, 'Those codes, and the expression of the individual genes are modifiable. The person you are right now is the result of the uncontrolled experiment of your life in which you have been bathing your genes with experience to give rise to the outcome of that experiment. If you don't like the results that make up your life thus far, you can change it at any time, whatever age' (cited in Holford, 2006).

I think the point we need to focus on here is that you can change it *at any age* – something which most of us probably don't realise. In fact, something like cancer is only 5% inherited and 95% life. So, we all know that we should eat better and live more healthily, don't we? Well, the answer according to a 2004 survey of 37,000 found that only 6% were in the optimum health category, with 44% in either the poor or very poor category (according to Patrick Holford's 2004 ONUK Survey).

The Western answer to pain is prescribed man-made drugs (NSAIDs), which are only relatively safe for short-term use, as gut bleeds, nausea, vomiting, headaches, and dizziness are all possible side effects. So what can you do instead of popping a painkiller every time you get a headache? Just head to your kitchen. That's right; you can turn your kitchen into a pharmacy. Personally, I grew up with a kitchen full of herbs and vitamins as the norm, so step inside mine and I'll show you around.

Get In Your Garden

I love my new greenhouse, which was crafted by our carpenter in situ in my garden. It is absolutely bulging with vegetables, some fruit, and some herbs. Food combining is the key. For example, berries are more potent protectors if combined with green veggies, mushrooms, and onions. This wonderfully healthy diet fuels the human genome's self-protective properties, and mixing the most powerfully protective foods helps to prevent cell damage that can lead to cancer, heart disease, and dementia, and kills heavily damaged cells. Two papers on this subject that might be of interest are *Fruit and veg intake in relation to risk of breast cancer in the black women's health study* (Boggs, Palmer and Wise et al., 2010) and *Cancer prevention with natural compounds* (Gullet, Amin and Bayraker et al., 2010).

My herbs and spices rack houses my favourite pain relieving and anti-inflammatory spices and herbs: turmeric, cayenne pepper, chilli, and ginger, especially for migraines and heartburn, rosemary for nerves, muscles, and chronic headaches, sage for hurting muscles and sore throat, and parsley for arthritic pain. As a side note, turmeric is called ukon in Japan and jiang huang in China, as well as curcuma and Indian saffron.

I have a nice selection of herbal teas to hand – which are very warming during the winter months – as tea contains flavonoids such as pain killing quercetin. I have a particular weakness for Earl Grey, although I find that nettle tea helps with arthritic pain, peppermint is great for digestive pain, and chamomile reduces the stress of pain and is relaxing – I have it before I go to bed, as it's good for the stomach and for getting sleep. Jasmine is said to be the healthiest of all, as it has the most antioxidants, but all teas have flavonoids, which are good for preventing heart disease, strokes and cancer. Scientists from Rutgers University stated that teas closely representing green teas are less fermented and act as the most powerful antioxidants. Buddhist and Shinto priests actually drink tea to stay awake during long meditations.

If you like beer rather than tea, hop extract nearly matched ibuprofen in painkilling effects. Olives I adore, and they also have anti-inflammatory and pain killing properties closely related to ibuprofen. For gynaecological pain, gin and tonic, Chinese herbs, Vitex agnus-castus, black cohosh, dong quai and St Johns Wort can all help.

Personally, I know I do not grow enough vegetables and that my diet is not vitamin and mineral rich enough to sustain intense, long, stressful days working, hence I supplement my meals with essentials form USANA Health Sciences, following lectures at my old university by American founder, Professor Wentz. He shared a lot of research into the effects of boosting the right combination of foods with vitamin and mineral supplements in both animals and humans. At the time, we were working with a film producer who was interested in preventative health and we were going to see what we could do on the subject of nutrients in our Western diet and soil levels. However, we hit a major negative about exposing information the public may find unsettling, so it didn't happen.

Smoothies

I love my morning smoothie. I make one for my breakfast to give me energy for my running, cycling, or dance/fit class, although even if you're not about to do exercise, it's a great way to start the day. My favourite – which I have a lot – includes almond milk, a banana, and some raspberries or strawberries, and this particular type of smoothie is easy to digest, which is good for me if I'm running afterwards. Bananas are said to make more happy juice in the brain, so I always include one in my smoothies if I can. I may also add pineapples as they have bromelain, which aids digestive pains, as well as papaya, which has papain that does the same thing, and cherries which have anthocyanin, a painkiller.

Then, after sport or as a snack, I enjoy my veggie juices – they're full of carotenoids, which are strong antioxidants and which help prevent any form of chronic disease. Juicing really does get addictive; you can almost hear your cells calling out to thank you. I often rummage around in my greenhouse and fridge to find seasonal veggies and fruit to make a yummy cocktail, which is basically a turbo shot of nutrients. Not only is this secret elixir good for your cells and your inner health, but it also shows on the outside with shiny hair and glowing skin. Basically, it's a really good beauty product in a cup, and you get all sorts of extra health benefits: you can sleep better, you can run longer, you can have fewer cravings for sugary food, and personally, it helps me to work sixteen hour days when I would otherwise be tempted to snooze on the sofa in front of the fire.

If I am looking for a particular health angle, I mix up some recipes. For example, I add more celery if the person has a blood pressure problem. Generally, I use a lot of carrots, then add celery, apple and broccoli, before flavouring with berries, ginger, lime or orange. To this I then add wheat and barley grass, as well as algae for some of my juices – small amounts only, though, as they're an acquired taste.

As an example, here is one of my favourite juices:

- 3 carrots.
- 1 apple.
- ½ lime.
- Small broccoli sprout.
- 3 celery sticks.
- Teaspoon of barley grass.

If you like beetroot and have high blood pressure, try this one:

- 3 celery sticks.
- 2 beetroots.
- 3 carrots.
- Ginger.

Ginger is anti-viral, so it's great in winter months if you regularly suffer from colds. It is also good for nausea and has been used in folk medicine for years. Occasionally, I add dried seaweed (I used to collect it as a biologist) in small amounts as it is very rich in protein, as well as calcium, iodine, magnesium, folate, iron, vitamin A, cancer fighting phytoestrogens and so on. So, next time you get a whiff of seaweed washed up on the beach, you may look more kindly at it and its many essential nutrients.

I will often put the juiced pulp into a soup, and my Tao and Chinese cookery books talk about the importance of eating cooked food, especially if ill or elderly. Raw food has more nutrients, but it is harder to digest and actually takes more energy to digest it. Cooked food is less nutritious, but it is already partly broken down and so is easier to digest. Therefore, it's swings and roundabouts, and a mix of both is a good idea.

Other Healthy Foods

One of my favourite warming foods is sweet potato soup, and the history of the sweet potato is quite interesting. Records go back to 1605 when an Okinawan man bought a seedling back from Fujian, a nearby Chinese province. Here they suffered from terrible typhoons – four a year, in fact – which tore out rice paddy fields, but their life saving sweet potatoes prevailed. They are said to be rich in goodies: carotenoids, saponins and flavonoids, as well as being high in vitamins E and C.

I nearly always put garlic in my warm veggies and soups; it is an age old healer and grows in my greenhouse, so it's easy for me to add to my food. Romans – as well as soldiers in and before World War One – used it in poultices to prevent infection from wounds, as it is good for the immune and cardiovascular systems and is also anti-cancer. Another anti-cancer food is onion, again something which is great in soups. Onions are also rich in flavonoids and gives a nice flavour to otherwise dull soups. If you use parsley as a garnish on your soups, it will help water excretion, as it is rich in vitamins, especially A and C. I always have almonds to hand as a snack, as well as pine nuts, sunflower seeds, and a few raisins.

In summary, my winning formula for pain relief would be some olives and fish oils, nuts, eggs, onion and garlic, a couple of herbs in tea or in food like the ones above, and fresh raw fruit in a smoothie or green veg juice, as these contain antioxidants, vitamins C and E, Q10 and lipoic acid. There – you now have your very own pharmacy of potent painkillers for every problem. If you are having an arthritic flare up, avoid vegetable oil, gluten (wheat, rye, barley), cooking at high temperatures, soda – as sugar spikes are linked to osteoarthritis of the knee – trans fats and too many processed foods.

Drugs and Nutrient Absorption

I am always being asked by patients who take herbal teas and supplements what they are able to take now they have been prescribed a new drug. When this happens, I arm them with literature and suggest they discuss it with the consultant or GP that is medically responsible for them and their prescription; if your medic has nutritional training, they will be able to advise you on what the purpose of the drug was for and whether it was appropriate to self-medicate on natural herbs, vitamins, and minerals at the same time. Sometimes they work against each other, so you have to be careful.

I am not a GP and therefore not trained in the pharmacology of drugs. I have, however, had many lectures from nutritionists, and GPs who are also nutritionists and pharmacists. Also, I have taught and worked alongside many different experts in this field, so I know that it is extremely important to discuss any self-medication with your GP. Without this information, the correct questions may not come up and it may be, in your case, that extra supplements or dietary adjustments would not help your health. You must always check.

The debate about supplements still rages on. I take them and it is a personal choice based on the research available. It's all about true information and the freedom of choice to make an intelligent decision about your future health.

Blood Pressure Tablets

Blood pressure tablets are largely ACE (Angiotensin Converting Enzyme) inhibitors, and they work on a substance in your kidney called rennin. This is converted to angiotensin I then angiotension II, the latter of which constricts blood vessels, raising BP (blood pressure) and releasing aldosterone, which adds sodium to increase loading on the heart. The enzyme responsible for this chain reaction is blocked by the drug – I remember this from all my biochemistry lectures at university. If you're on blood pressure tablets, you can talk with your consultant regarding the safety of taking supplements. For example, ask them if it would be OK to take coenzyme Q10 or B6. If you wish to get further expert advice, see a nutritional consultant with your GP's approval.

B Blockers

These slow the heart by blocking the sinus rhythm, and also lower BP over time. This depletes Q10, which is a shame because this guy plays a key role in our cardiovascular systems. Heart failure drugs that contain digoxin also deplete B vitamins, calcium, magnesium, and phosphate.

Diuretics

Diuretics remove extra fluid, and they are often used in combination with ACE inhibitors for people with high BP. The amount of urine is increased and there is a vitamin depletion, especially zinc, calcium, magnesium, potassium, vitamin B1, vitamin B6, folic acid, coenzyme Q10, and phosphate.

Cholesterol Drugs

Most common cholesterol drugs feature statins, which bind cholesterol in the gut, blocking absorption. In several articles I've found, they talk of a reduction in coenzyme Q10, folic acid, vitamins D, E, and A, and carotenoids. If your GP/consultant/nutritionist suggests it is OK for you to supplement, make sure you don't take it at the same time as the drug, as it will bind them too.

Antibiotics

Antibiotics cannot distinguish between friendly gut flora and unfriendly bacteria, and they deplete nutrients such as vitamins B, D, and K, magnesium, calcium, potassium, zinc, copper, and iron. Consult a medic with nutritionist knowledge or a qualified nutritionist for more information. Antifungal tablets deplete calcium, potassium, and magnesium. Anti-viral also deplete nutrients, the popular ones which are listed being potassium, magnesium, phosphorus, calcium, vitamin B12, carnitine, copper, and zinc (Fowles, 2003).

Diabetic Drugs

This disease needs a healthy diet full of antioxidant properties. Drugs will deplete certain nutrients such as B12, folic acid, and Q10. Get an expert involved.

Anti-Inflammatory Drugs

These are available in several forms, the most common being NSAID, which are non-steroidal and cost the NHS £250 million a year. They block pain by cutting off the body's anti-inflammatory response, however, they should only be used for short periods of time due to the side effects (Allison et al., 1984).

Did you know that Willow tree bark is an anti-inflammatory and therefore a natural form of aspirin? Aspirin – which is a derivative of willow tree bark – is often the first drug employed to relieve pain and inflammation, and it is also known for its blood thinning abilities in nature. Nowadays, patients are advised to have a mild dosage, as it can be toxic if it is too high; too much aspirin gives early signs of ringing in the ears and gastric irritation. I remember that years ago, everyone thought it was the best thing since sliced bread. Then, back in 1980, the world nutrition congress stirred up a hornet's nest by saying that one aspirin can cause gut bleeding for a week, and that it also slows down cartilage growth. It can also destroy vitamin C, which is needed for collagen, so if it is being used to treat arthritic pain, long-term use is bad news.

Our poor cells are always under attack, receiving hits all the time – scientists actually came up with a figure of at least 127 per day, which is incredible. Damage comes from radiation, viruses, and bacteria and toxins from foods. Beyond damaging the functionality of the cell, these hits can turn on tumour promoting genes or turn off tumour suppressing genes. Hormones then kick in to feed the cancers – unless you live in a small group of Japanese islands like the Okinawans, of course.

Low calorie diets reduce the incidence of cancer, and Western diets are 40% greater than healthy Eastern diets (Weindruch and Sohal, 1997). It is known that a good diet helps with cancer prevention (Baranowski and Stables, 2000), and between five and seven portions of fruit and vegetables every day boosts vitamins, minerals, flavonoids, and fibres.

NSAIDs are only relatively safe for short-term use, and are not useful firefighting drugs for long-term use for anything, as your doctor will explain. In some patients, they may cause not only gut bleeds, but also nausea, vomiting, headaches, or dizziness. Some chronic arthritic conditions have long-term drugs prescribed for them, and a qualified expert may discuss mineral depletions, which can include calcium, vitamin C, potassium, magnesium, zinc, folic acid, selenium, and iron. Methotrexate is often used for my rheumatoid patients, and for people with cancer. You must check with your consultant and qualified nutritionist if taking supplements, because they can interfere with drugs. For example, folic acid is depleted for a reason in this case.

Hormone Replacement Therapy

I see a lot of ladies who struggle with their arthritis flaring up at times of menopause or hysterectomies. Some take natural dietary advice from nutritional experts, some use progesterone creams, and others use hormone replacement therapy (HRT). The latter suits a lot of ladies, but certainly not all. Consult a doctor who has a keen interest in women's health issues and nutrition, and see if supplementing with minerals and B vitamins is advised. Chinese medicine and herbs can also help – I have seen that both in my clinics and in clinics in the East – and always keep your GP in the loop with what you are taking.

Physiotherapists and doctors, if you are reading this and are interested in women's health, you should go on a nutritional and/or acupuncture course. I have a friend (Jon Hobbs, AACP director, lecturer and physiotherapist) who currently runs accredited courses in acupuncture for women's health problems (see appendix for contact details). Just another plug about exercise now, ladies: bones dem bones dem dry bones... more than ever we need resistive exercises to help with oestrogen reduction and ageing.

The Contraceptive Pill

When treating headaches and migraines, I am often asked about the effect of the pill on them, as well as if the patient should alter their diet or start taking any supplements. I understand from colleagues that it is beneficial to have a good diet and to consider a multi vitamin/mineral complex rich in B vitamins, as well as food containing tryptophan and tyrosine. I urge you to discuss it with your GP and someone who has studied nutrition in-depth. I enjoy studying women's health, and in my next book I will go into more detail, touching on Dr. Northrup's wonderful bible, *Women's Bodies, Women's Wisdom* (Piatkus, 2009).

Depression

A lot of my patients who come to the clinic to see myself or my colleagues are depressed due to chronic pain and disability. Statistics say that 20% of arthritis sufferers also suffer from depression, although I think it must be higher. If your GP agrees, discuss your condition with a well-qualified nutritionist; it is a good idea to look at making your diet healthier, and if appropriate, supplement with B vitamins and Q10. A close friend's daughter suffered for many years and reacted badly to all her drugs. In recent years, she has had a personal trainer and has started training every day, as well as drinking juices and smoothies. With a good diet and expert advice, she is better than ever, which is great to hear.

Asthma

A long time ago at Birmingham University, I did some research into asthma; I took pictures of mast cells and investigated how triggering the membrane resulted in an explosion of histamine and chemical cascades that reap havoc. Then, years later, as an on call physiotherapist at the hospitals, I would get in the car at 2 or 3 a.m. and go off to help with tight-chested, breathless souls. As a kid, I took part in a research trial for hay fever, as I used to be a big time sufferer in the summer; I had injections that would make my arm swell up greatly, and following that, I experienced asthma. I didn't mind being a guinea pig, though, as hopefully that meant a poor animal wouldn't have to be experimented on.

I was lucky that my asthma was never severe, and I had the blue and brown puffers until – through exercise and diet – I was able to throw them away, and asthma has never darkened my doors since. I learnt, however, when I worked in asthma clinics, that I did not inhale the stuff properly, so if you use an inhaler, make sure you get a lesson, and get as healthy as you possibly can. A drug called theophylline depletes B vitamins, so as long as your doctor is happy, focus on having a good, healthy diet and taking multivitamins and mineral complexes that are rich in vitamin B.

Graham, a singer from Norwich, had steroids for his asthma for years, as he suffered badly and experienced severe side effects. He reads my health tips on Facebook, and although I haven't seen him sing in 25 years, I hear that – while fragile – he is still singing.

Parkinson's Disease

I have some dear patients with this cruel disease, and it affects both the mind and body; Parkinson's depletes the body of a brain neurotransmitter called dopamine, as the basal ganglia experience degenerative change. One patient had wires linked through his brain to a transducer, which stopped his hand tremors wonderfully, and I think stem cell research may come up with some good results one day. There are many drugs used for this disease, one of which is levodopa, which helps with dopamine. They do, however, deplete potassium and a protein which helps happiness. Of course, sometimes a drug may be necessary, and side effects are a small price to pay if the general quality of life is better. Always check with your consultant if you want to take supplements on top of drugs for Parkinson's.

I have cross referenced the nutrient depletions with (to name a few) Patrick Holford's lecture notes, Professor Wentz's lecture notes, Clell M Fowles' book, *Drugs And Nutrient Depletion* (DAC Health, 2003) and *Death by Prescription* by Ray Strand (Thomas Nelson, 2003).

Let me reiterate: if we had healthy, rich soils, all these vitamins and minerals would make the need for supplements unnecessary. However, we don't have nutrient-rich food, due to soil depletion, early harvesting, hybrids, added pesticides, and food storage techniques. A good book to read on this subject is by Dr Ray Strand and is called, *What Your Doctor Doesn't Know About Nutritional Medicine May Be Killing You* (Thomas Nelson, 2002). The USANA website has lots of links on this subject as well.

Cancer Drugs (Chemotherapy and Radiotherapy)

I have strong opinions on this subject, however, I do not feel it is appropriate to discuss this flippantly in a general manual, as it is too serious a subject. You can get info snippets on my Facebook pages if you wish to know more and I will revisit this area in my next book, *The Human Garage*. However, I have a learned friend in this field who is nearly qualified in naturopathic nutrition and works in my practice currently as a highly qualified physiotherapist, called Pam, so I'll be calling upon her expertise in the next book.

Adverse Drug Reactions

The Journal of the American Medical Association wrote the infamous report on adverse drug reactions: in 1994, 2.2 million people went to hospital due to a reaction to a drug, and 106,000 consequently died (Lazarou, Pomeranz, and Corey, cited in JAMA, 1998). Heart disease killed 743,000 each year, cancer 529,000, strokes 150,000, and road traffic accidents 41,000, with 100,000 deaths being caused by properly prescribed drugs and 80,000 by improperly prescribed drugs. So, that's 180,000 deaths due to drugs in total (Cullen, Bates, Laird et al., cited in JAMA, 1995). Get my point? Hence the importance of preventative health to get you as well as you can be to have the best outcome from the help of drugs.

So, let's recap: in the USA, the number one cause of death is heart disease, the runner up is cancer, third drugs, fourth strokes, then finally – with a lot less – road traffic accidents. It makes you think, doesn't it?

Healthy Food for Our Lungs

On a more serious note, we can look at the key to healthy breathing by looking at some good nosh that will help combat breathing problems. Our clinic is near to a forest, and while the trees don't stand between us and the road, they do help filter pollution from all of the cars passing by. Recently, there was a programme about how it was scientifically proven that trees filter out some of the rubbish we breathe in. So, on my own land – where the council allows us to do so – I am planting some more, as it concerns me that our lungs will tell a story of the roads we live and work by. On a personal note, as a student, and often making do with a less than perfect diet, I picked up every chest infection going on the wards. Today, I still usually succumb to an episode of bronchitis in the winter, though it rarely lasts with my healthy eating and the supplements I take.

Healthy foods for our lungs are rich in substances called cytokines and mediators, to help control inflammatory cells, as well as omega oils, vitamin C, and antioxidants, all of which are essential (Moldoveanu, 2008).

These foods include yellow, orange, and red fruit and veggies, carrots, red peppers, squash, watermelon, tomatoes (carotenoids), broccoli, cabbage, and cauliflower. Sulforaphane rids bacteria and helps protect against cancer, so I always have oodles of homemade soups in the winter bubbling away on the hearth. Beans, sprouts, and onions give a good flavour, though they don't always agree with digestion and you may need bricks on your duvet! I take apples into work as they are rich in antioxidants (quercetin), and in fact, all fruits in my smoothies are rich in flavonoids and plant pigments, as well as being anti-inflammatory, antimutagenic, and anticarcinogenic. On another note, if you're anything like me, you'll be pleased to know that nice, warming cups of tea are excellent for the chest.

Hair Health

My grandma always used to brush my hair, telling me that our general health and vitality shows in how healthy our locks are, so make sure your soups and dinners contain these foods if your hair is looking unkempt and needs love. I have long hair and I swim a lot, but I keep it healthy by focusing on these foods. I buy from our local farm shop as well as picking some of these ingredients from my garden. Here is your hair medicine:

- Sweet potatoes. These are rich in goodies, and I love them roasted or mashed, or – in moderation – in a juicer (B carotene and vitamin A).
- Spinach (folate, vitamin C, B carotene, plus iron).
- Cauliflower (B5 pantothenic acid).
- Kale, broccoli, tomatoes, avocados, legumes, lentils.
- Free range eggs (biotin, vitamin B).
- Fish protein (omega 3, zinc).
- Fruit, e.g. apples (vitamin C).

Herbs

Before I talk more about herbs, can I just say that herbal therapies are to be taken seriously – they are natural drugs, but they are still real drugs with real side effects. In Germany alone, £4 billion is spent each year on herbs (Klepser and Klepser, 1999).

I grew up with herbs used as medicine. However, as Dr Strand echoes in his book, *Death By Prescription*, they are nature's drugs but they can actually interact with prescribed drugs. For example, liquorice root can stimulate aldosterone release and can cause cardiac problems if used at high doses over time. In Germany, they recommend a break at six weeks. St John's Wort with black cohosh could lead to a miscarriage, and St John's Wort and Prozac can increase serotonin and can lead to headaches, confusion, and irritability.

Ginkgo biloba is known for improving circulation, however, it also thins blood, so when used with aspirin, it could cause serious complications (Roundtree, 1999). I find supplements of glucosamine sulphate great for joints and I take a small dosage daily. I have had only one patient allergic to it (and fish oils), and his chest pain had him rushed off to hospital. Out of 10,000 patients, that's the only scary story I've heard, but one is enough to elicit caution (Reginster et al., 2001).

Used wisely, herbs are inspiring, and the regular ones in my kitchen garden are a great source of antioxidants. Now, let's lighten the subject; I am feeling far too serious writing all of the above.

Romantic Herbs

Here's a more cheerful use for herbs, rather than illness. Returning to your herb kitchen garden and spell book, you can create a special lusty cocktail which is meant to get the juices going on Valentine's night, as well as allowing you to forget your aches and pains. Here goes the strange recipe: a mug of oat straw, salty seaweed, earthy burdock root, sweet scented rose petals, and dark chocolate. It doesn't sound very tasty to me, but I'll let you make your own mind up! Then, historically, lovers decorate their house and self with sprigs of rosemary, lavender, and basil... very strange, but who knows, it might work!

Potted Rosemary has been used as a sign of romantic love for centuries, with sprigs being worn by brides in the middle ages. These sprigs were planted out afterwards, and if they grew it showed a strong relationship. Sprigs were also planted with potential lovers' names, to see which grew stronger. That's where I went wrong – I didn't do the sprig test! Lavender sprigs are also used as an aphrodisiac. In a similar vein, basil pots can be placed outside eligible women's homes, as basil means commitment and fertility, and in Romania it means the same as an engagement ring – much cheaper too.

Women's Problems

Can diet help with women's problems? Yes, actually. A lot of my middle aged female patients get aching joints around period times and menopause, and diet is so important to help this and keep joints healthy in general. Interestingly, my Chinese tutors told me that Chinese herbs play a key role in this, so if you're getting particularly bad stomach cramps and pain, try Vitex agnus-castus, dong quai, chamomile, and St Johns Wort, or black cohosh for the menopause, just to name a few key ones.

Avoiding Digestive/Reflux Problems

I have an acidic stomach and when my alkaline ioniser works, it really eases any acidity. Get yourself a pH stick, and eat more alkaline foods. Risks for mouth, oesophagus, colon, and rectum cancer are a lack of fruit and veg, very hot drinks, too much alcohol, and smoking. Preventative measures are a good diet, especially foods including vitamin A and C and selenium.

As I've mentioned, I always have green veggies in my juicer, and mix in green algae, wheat and barley grass. Studies demonstrate that green vegetable consumption is an excellent way to eat us into health (Fuhrman, 2010). I consider my greenhouse to be a living, breathing medicine cabinet – and I'd have been burnt at the stake for saying that years ago! However, it's now been found that the populations with the highest intake of healthy vegetables live longer and healthier lives (Li, Ford, and Zhao et al., 2010).

I actually took photographs of my vibrantly colourful veggies this year, and this vibrancy hides secrets to our immunity, with a thousand or more specific phytochemicals hidden inside. These guys are potent homes to anti-oxidants, whose roles are to attack extra free radicals that have over spilled into areas they shouldn't be in, attacking healthy tissue.

It's a sobering thought that 2kg of us is bacteria. In fact, the biologist in me knows that one type climbed inside our cells and is actually our powerhouse, called mitochondria. These are tricky little guys: without good nutrition, they don't kill cancer cells and fire up fibromyalgia. We evolved alongside bacteria and we have 100 trillion bacteria in our garbage department – our digesting gut. Nice thought, right? I could never understand why we had the play pen put next to the garbage outlet, but anyway, moving on… Health promoting bacteria fight naughty bacteria as well as fungi and viruses. I don't eat meat but I still drink some pasteurised milk and both of these carry the less desirable Streptococcus. My love of veggies boosts the friendly Lactobacillus acidophilus and Bifidobacteria. Also, I am not a baby cow, so why do I want to have lots of milk to potentially make me grow big and fat? You don't see humans hanging off cows' udders in fields…

If you are prone to getting indigestion and irritable bowels, have a few of these in your cupboard: peppermint oil, for example, is a great antispasmodic. I love my alkaline ioniser and I avoid too much in the way of acidic food. Linseed is a natural anti-inflammatory, and slippery elm coats the walls of the stomach, protecting us from toxins and irritants. Pectin – a gel from fruit – takes out more toxins, and fennel and fenugreek are great and lovely on a salad. Acacia gum and alfalfa cleanse, blessed thistle and milk thistle detox, and cloves and red clover are anaesthetic, anti-inflammatory, and antispasmodic. If you are suffering with digestive problems, these types of food are kind for you: grains, fish, olive oil, nuts, and seeds. Drink lots of water and herbal teas – personally, I have a whole cupboard full.

Any oil including olive oil is full of empty calories at 120 calories per tablespoon. Eat nuts and seeds instead – it is associated with weight loss due to the fact the oils and fats do not get stored in us in the same way that the likes of olive oil does (Fuhrman, 2011). Nuts are a great source of protein, and don't forget, green veg is 50% healthy, alkaline protein. Animal protein if in excess is stored as fat, and in the process rapes calcium and phosphates from the bones to reduce acidity. I don't consume red meat so that's one less thing for me to have to work on.

Getting Good Sleep

Apart from addressing the root cause of any mental stress, what we eat and when – as well as how sugary or stimulating the food is – all play a role in how well we sleep. Sleep is a key to health, as it is whilst we snooze that our body repairs itself and stores away memory as we dream. I drink herbal teas if I have been writing far too late in my study at home, as they contain a variety of herbs, valerian root, magnesium citrate, GABA, inositol, lemon balm, 5-HTP, serotonin, melatonin, L-Theanine, hops, and passion flower. All of these things help get you sleepy before bed, and personally, I put quieter music on and do a few gentle yoga stretches. Don't have lots of dark chocolate, as it has caffeine in it, although it does pick me up if I'm on a long, late drive and don't want to sleep and die! If you're trying to sleep, however, avoid acidic citrus foods, and have no mustard, spices, or cakes – as you'll need to avoid sugar spikes.

Here's some unusual foods that you may not know can help you sleep: you can enjoy bananas, as they have tryptophan in them, which converts to serotonin happy juice in the brain, as well as magnesium, potassium, and melatonin. Tart cherry juice also has melatonin in it, and almond butter contains magnesium. All of these foods will help you on your way to a sound sleep, something we must all get enough of if we are to stay healthy.

Foods That Age Us

None of us want to look our age, but instead of going down the surgery route, why not take a look at your diet instead? What you're eating could be adding to your premature ageing, making you look your age as well as feeling it. Too much sugar leads to chronic inflammation, and everyone can be guilty of this, even me – who doesn't love a little bit of chocolate now and then? Trans fats and deep frying, on the other hand, are extremely unhealthy and I avoid these completely. Processed foods add to cancer and premature ageing, as the nutrition is stripped out and sugar and salt added, as well as artificial products, which all age us. I love raw salads and veggies, thank goodness, although I wasn't so keen when I was a kid.

Milk that is pasteurised kills off digestive enzymes and makes 50% of calcium unusable. I drink your semi-skimmed regular stuff, as well as soya and almond. I grew up on lots of milk and it's sad to hear that it's not all as good as I was led to believe. Sunflower oil and corn has too much omega 6 and not enough omega 3. You should avoid all aspartame sweeteners. One glass of alcohol a night is good for you, but two plus is ageing. Red wine in small amounts is anti-ageing, whiskey is blood thinning and pain relieving, and gin and tonic (quinine) can be used as a muscle relaxant for pain.

Anti-Ageing Foods

Berries have phytonutrients and antioxidants, so pop them in your smoothie – I do when I can get hold of them. Garlic and green veggies – especially spinach – are great in your soups and dinners, and proteins (ideally organic) are also good anti-ageing foods. Omega 3 oil foods and food supplements with vitamin E help protect against radical damage.

I don't have degrees in nutrition, however, I have walked with shamans in their jungles and have a rudimentary knowledge that, for most of us, is lost. Furthermore, I have been spoilt with inspiring lectures from many people, including several from Patrick Holford, whose books are a library in themselves! I don't have space to go into further detail on foreign herbs – as this is just a taster of healthy ideas – but I must mention Ayurvedic herbs. With these, the whole plant is used to avoid side effects, but in Western herbal medicine, only the active ingredient is used. Ayurvedic medicine draws on 50 herbs and fruits picked at a certain time and then cooked for a certain time, and goes well beyond my basic home pharmacy. Chinese medicine is the combination of using herbs and acupuncture, and again the herbs are mixed precisely. Now, I have to note here that some of the medicine was taken inappropriately from animals, and that part I cannot condone. Before the authorities condoned Chinese medicine, we did have some in my clinic with great effect, and patients found it beneficial to combine the acupuncture with herbs.

Losing Weight the Right Way

One of my patients, Joan, runs a local division of a well-known slimming club. Joan has been concerned about her weight all of her life, and therefore has gone on many, many diets over the years, from calorie counting to the latest fad. When she came to see me, I looked at her fibromyalgia and investigated (with the help of a nutritionist) the nutrition she needed because of this condition, changing her diet so she could eat healthy food, but food that was specific to the fibromyalgia. Mainly, I made it more alkaline, and she lost ten pounds in a week. This just shows that certain people need certain things more than others, and that it isn't always about simply cutting down your calorie intake or choosing smaller portions of food. It's all about knowing what's good for you and sticking to it – you don't need fad diets or to starve yourself to get to a healthy weight.

Food Intolerances

Modern lifestyles have led to an explosion of obesity, diabetes, heart conditions, cancer, and osteoarthritis, to name just a few. Obesity, diabetes, and liver damage are all closely linked to glycaemic load, and this can be measured with a blood test at our clinic. The analysis is then done at YorkTest (a food intolerance and allergy testing company). A liver check test is also available.

Homocysteine can similarly be analysed. Most people in the UK have never heard of homocysteine and are unaware that it is the most important predictor of many degenerative diseases, such as heart disease, stroke, and peripheral artery disease. Basically, it is a product converted mostly by animal protein, and healthy bodies break it down into harmless products.

You can get tested for this (see the YorkTest in the appendix) and some doctors believe it to be a much better indicator than cholesterol levels; a homocysteine level above 13 has been shown to predict 67% of all deaths within five years. A quick blood test is all that is needed for you to find out how much at risk you are. With the Okinawa project, as some of the youngsters began to eat a Westernised diet, their homocysteine level rose, and with it, circulatory disease (Gey and Alfthan, 1997). With the same genes and a different diet, cardiovascular disease also appeared (Willcox, Willcox, Suzuki, and Todoriki, 2000).

Around 45% of UK residents suffer from some form of food intolerance, which can manifest itself either rapidly, such as with a peanut allergy, or more slowly, with symptoms such as IBS, pain after eating, eczema, or asthma. A comprehensive food intolerance test is available, which will analyse your tolerance to 113 foods.

Percy's Story

Percy was a 25 stone Italian musician with back ache, or stenosis of his lumbar spine, to be precise. In a nutshell, Percy explained his story to me: "Help me, I am in such pain in my back and down my leg, but I'm scared about having surgery and having time off work. My brother came to my Christmas orchestral performance, felt ill, and went home – dying at just 50 years old. The doctor said it was a blood clot that travelled into his heart and it would have been quick, just like my dad's death." He said that with a family genetically predisposed to high cholesterol and fatty arteries, his obesity was a big nail in his coffin.

He continued. "Help me! I am 49. I have a gifted life ahead of me playing the cello and singing with my orchestra, but I am homesick for my Italian life and food. I have been comfort eating a lot of naughty food and I cannot give it up, as it's my way of giving myself a treat. I love my food and I cannot diet – I get too upset. However, my brother's death has scared me, and I'm not sure I would make it through the surgery."

Well, I went to one of his performances, sitting and watching his very rotund, stooped figure wrapped around his cello – he mirrored its shape. The audience was spellbound and the conductor drove the orchestra into a frenzy of vibrant music; he was definitely gifted. However, being that big, he was digging his grave with his teeth.

I got it. He associated healthy food with a painful experience and saw unhealthy food as a short-term, pleasurable, loving act. I used some NLP techniques and introduced an alkalising diet, after buying him a juicer. I then gave him my favourite delicious recipes, and 'hardwired' him to feel pleasure and love for his body and life with this new food blended into his existing diet. The new rush of vitamins and minerals, alkalising veggie juices, and wheatgrass/barley grass drinks reset his taste buds, pain-free. I told him to say some mantras out loud as he drank, and eating healthy food strengthened his resolve. His previously acidic body stopped hanging onto fat cells, and his new metabolism started saving his life, without taking anything away from him – get my point?

Percy lost five stone very easily and started craving healthy food and reducing his intake of unhealthy food. His diet had to start prior to my IMS (dry needling techniques) as I could not operate through his fat. Once his weight allowed his cells to function more healthily, the MRT (magnetic resonance treatment) regenerated his discogenic material and reduced the inflammatory problem around his trapped nerve and arthrosis facet joint. Pilates restored his core and he was able to begin a pain-free, longer life. Percy no longer had any need for what would have been life threatening surgery in his unhealthy condition. All he needed to do was listen to his body and change the fuel he was giving it.

Too Unhealthy to Ride a Horse

Bertie Brown loved her horse, Eric, and she had ridden him for many a year, until now. She explained to me that with her recent husband's passing, she had been comfort eating and she now had really bad hip pain and stiffness. Due to her obesity and inability to throw her leg over Eric, she could no longer ride him.

Bertie had OA in her hips, accelerated and compounded by the four stone she had put on over the last couple of years. Also, she now had a drugs cabinet for all her tablets: blood pressure, statins, diuretics (water tablets), arthritis tablets, pills to stop her gut reacting to pills... you name it, she had it. Her diet was full of fast food and carbohydrates – and lots of it – and she had taken to baking lots of sponge cakes. Her kitchen was a disaster zone; she said she couldn't bear eating alone, so she went out a lot or snacked on unhealthy, sugary food. This made her feel some short-term comfort.

I took her to the market and bought fresh veggies, then went online and got her a juicer. While we were out, she had to stop a lot to lean on her stick, as she hadn't commenced her prescribed exercises, and was consequently unfit and out of breath. I went on the USANA site and advised her on talking to their medics about essential vitamins and minerals.

As an aside, whilst in America, I got my husband, Alan, to research the CIA files on vitamin and mineral products and the companies that sell them – the data is not available in the UK. All I will say is that from the data, we found there was a lot of proof that fresh products grown in rich, fertile soil and eaten soon after is not a Western experience. Many diseases are connected to nutrient deficiencies. Vitamins and minerals from this company (USANA) came highly recommended, and after meeting the fascinating Professor Wentz – the founder and owner of USANA, as well as a brilliant scientist – I was convinced.

Anyway, I digress. I suggested that she should invest in nutritional advice and talk with her GP about heading down this avenue, but when I came back a week later to a pantry full of the fruit and veg I had bought, an unopened box of tablets, and a grumpy, unridden horse, I didn't feel so smart, I can tell you.

"Do you love your horse?" I asked, exasperated at her. "Yes I do," she replied, "and it's breaking my heart not to ride him." I had a light bulb moment then and did some NLP over a cup of earl grey tea. "Not breaking your heart enough to do anything about it," I said untactfully, and she got angry, because she had no tools in the box to do anything about it. I got inside her head and I made her shrink down a picture of a slice of cake and enlarge one of her riding her horse. Then, I placed pictures of her on horseback in her healthy cupboard, and pictures of an empty field in her cupboards full of junk food. Get my point?

It is always good to give the tools before changing anything, so we started straight away, as if you cannot see a way out, your animal instinct will make you bear your teeth. Give a meaningful purpose, and by doing this, change can happen – it just depends on priority and commitment. I don't like going to someone's bedside when it's too late and being asked to kill them because their cells are too sick to recover and the pain too much to bear. This is a time when most people are prepared to change, but it's too late.

Anyway, Bertie lost her disease, changed her eating habits, and came to my clinic to have hip treatment to resolve her hip problem. No longer needing drugs, she lost four stone and Eric got ridden, all not quite in a day's work.

Focusing on Preventative Health

In summary, the truth is that nutritional science has made phenomenal discoveries in recent years, and if you apply this relatively new science to the West, its impact on diet should shape up the rapidly deteriorating health destiny due to obesity and chronic degenerative disease. We talked about needing a good immune system and a good source of unrefined plant products to achieve this. We also spoke of poor diets in the West and Americans achieving only 5% intake of healthy veg, so there is lots of room to improve your life's longevity and general health.

Our marketing is aimed at a belief system that equates a long, healthy, pain-free life with medicine, shots, diagnostic tests, more drugs, and surgery. Nothing could be further from the truth. A report from the Kaiser foundation stated that at least one third of medical spending was actually making people sicker. Until both a belief system in preventative health and taking responsibility for your own health is firmly in place, we are all on very shaky ground. As I said, only 2% of world health care funds is spent on preventative health, which is staggering when you think of all the disease statistics. For example, 37% of women and 44% of men will endure cancer in their lifetime. That's nearly every third woman and every other man.

If – like me – you are female and want to stay slim, you should be eating between 1,400 and 1,800 calories a day. Only 150 of those should be animal products or refined carbohydrates. Boys, between 1,800 and 2,400 and ideally only 200 calories of naughty stuff. The good news is that at last some of the top chefs in the world are cooking healthily, providing great tasting, immune supporting, cancer and degenerative disease preventing nosh (Fuhrman, 2010).

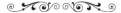

Once you've read this chapter, please go to page 248 of the appendix and complete the traffic light questionnaire for nutrition and hydration again to see how you have improved.

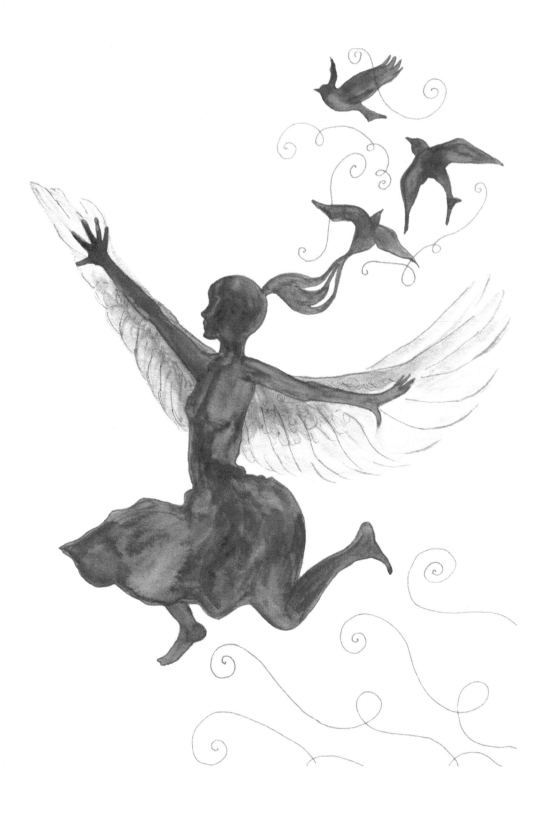

Fitness

This life is yours
Take the power
to choose what you want to do
and do it well
Take the power
to love what you want in life
and love it honestly
Take the power
to walk in the forest
and be a part of nature
Take the power
to control your own life
No one else can do it for you
Take the power
to make your life
healthy
exciting
worthwhile
and very happy

– Susan Polis Schutz

Before you read this chapter, please go to page 251 of the appendix and complete the traffic light questionnaire for fitness.

Note: For exercises described in this chapter, please see the appendix on page 257 for a complete list of images and names.

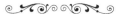

*T*oday I find that humans are far too sedentary, all too often sitting in front of a computer by day, followed by sitting in front of a TV at night. This lack of physical activity causes emotional and physiological imbalances, but we can change this by looking at how we exercise; improving your fitness changes your chemistry, acts as a powerful antidepressant, promotes mental clarity, and reduces the likelihood of cancer.

If you're not happy with either how you look or feel about your weight, then with correct guidance, you can break out of inactivity and be rewarded by smiling at yourself whenever you see your reflection. I will guide you, showing you how you can learn more about how and when you should exercise, as getting the correct mix can extend your life.

When I am working at my clinic, I hear echoing around the walls: I am too old to exercise, too old to work. Are you too old to exercise? Well, no one told Jiroemon Kimura (born 1897) that he was too old. He passed away recently at age 116, farming until he was 90 years old. Remember the *Carry On* films? Well, did you know that Barbara Windsor carries on exercising in her late 70s? You can find her in her gym wear keeping fit outside in Hyde Park.

Over 450,000 people in the USA and over 70,000 people in the UK risk total knee replacement every year. Want to talk pain? Then talk TKR. What's worse is that it is unsuccessful 10% of the time, and you can even die from having total knee replacement. Furthermore, the age for TKR is constantly dropping. Why? Anybody want to hazard a guess? That's right: obesity. Now, this isn't proven yet, but it is most likely the biggest cause.

So, what happens when you get fat? Ladies, take the 'C' off chips and you know what you get! Guys, you put it on around the waist and lose sight of your favourite toy! What you probably don't know is that your knees are loaded with up to four times your weight, so every extra stone (14 lbs) is an extra four stone (56 lbs) on your knees – that's why knees are so often the first casualty with OA. If you want to know why the four times multiple occurs, it's because of leverage. Now, you are intelligent people, and you are surely interested in health or you wouldn't be here. So, why have you made the decision to get arthritis? Made the decision to get lots of pain? Made the decision to risk surgery and even death? It's because much of the pain associated with the pleasure of eating too much is too far away, and anyway, going to the gym is a pain for most. We need to change the way we think about exercise, and hopefully this chapter will go some way to doing that for you.

Here's some more cheery news: an in-depth study into retirement found that men in their sixties are every bit as good at driving business than those physically and mentally in their prime. In later life, prescriptive exercise is more effort than swallowing a pill, but it is well worth it; in a nutshell, you get less senility and less pain. Exercise weaves its magic, strengthening the heart, releasing more neurotransmitters for cell communication, boosting BDNF for improving neural connections in the brain, aiding metabolism, improving blood flow, stimulating toxic disposal systems, and strengthening bones.

This next fact gets me out running in howling gales and rain: current research in Sweden shows that exercise alters the way genes work in the tissue that stores fat, and changes in adipose tissue storage sites were measurable even with just two workouts a week. Epigenetics has always fascinated me since studying biology, and this is the study of how chemical alterations will change how genes work in a cell. This allows us to fine tune our body to a changing environment.

Exercise alters this process in muscle cells and improves how sugar is processed. Furthermore, adipose tissue (fat cells) is an organ in its own right, producing active chemicals that have profound effects on the body. In this tissue, 18,000 markers were found on 7,663 genes! This is leading to a greater understanding of why exercise helps fatty tissue do its job properly, which means that as we get older, we don't have to have such a lumpy, bumpy body. This smooth body needs a good structural support.

Exercise Your Bones, dem bones dem bones dem old bones

Bones are remodelled throughout their life, as they respond to stresses put on them by activity, and every day, millions of old bone cells get replaced by new ones. Fibres within the bone matrix – that act like bridge girders – need weight bearing exercise to trigger reactions at connecting stress points. This triggers a cascade of biochemical reactions which, in turn, stimulates bone growth. In space, weightlessness cannot trigger bone matrix repair and bones thin. Remember the film *Gravity*? Sandra Bullock had wobbly legs when she landed from space. George Clooney gives me wobbly legs, but that's a whole other story…

In the same way as being in space, running, cycling, and swimming is not enough to reverse osteoporotic changes. In one study of mature ladies, a year of aerobic exercise resulted in an average of 4% bone loss. Weight building exercises took two years to reverse the loss. The American College of Sports medicine and the Osteoporosis Society (to name just two) insist on the prescription of aerobic exercise to include weights. Did you know? Just three hours of immobilisation, and we start to rot. Disuse means death. Don't be a couch potato.

Exercise is vital for healthy ageing, so get out of that chair! When we slouch in our chairs, we don't breathe correctly, we have less lung capacity, less oxygen, a poorer blood flow, a weaker heart, and less nutrient delivery. Smooth muscles tighten up to take up the slack, and our blood pressure readings go up. Blood flow can't accommodate sudden movements anymore, so dizziness follows, and with it, increased accidents. Men's sexual potency falls, the gut slows, and digestion fails. Sugar metabolism struggles and diabetes is more likely to take hold. In an article in Psychological Medicine, Dregan and M.C Gulliford wrote about how intense exercise helps brain function (Dregan & Gulliford, 2013), so you can remember where you put your gym wear! Get my drift?

Here are some more facts I sourced for you to back up reasons to exercise – for all you academic buffs out there. Whether you are old or young, 'it's widely acknowledged that a healthy body equals a healthy mind. The government recommends a minimum of 150 minutes of exercise per week, between the ages of 19 and 64' (Dregan, 2013). A word to the wise – if you don't exercise at all, start. If you are new to exercise, start small and just walk a little further than usual. Exercise doesn't have to mean enduring lengthy, intense programmes or taking up a gym membership, although I think the discipline of going and the social angle is great. If you are exercising on your own, you still need to add in working out with weights as well as aerobic exercise, such as walking.

Did you know that at 44 years old, without exercising, we are at the peak depressive age? However, at 70 – if we follow a fitness programme – it is possible to be as physically fit and happy as we were when we were 20! Another study got a group of 60 year olds to start doing three long swims a week, and their medical measurements and tests were those of 40 year olds.

Exercise is much like medicine – it doesn't have to taste nice, but the outcome is more than worth it. Being disciplined about getting your exercise is your key to longevity, so exercise regularly and effectively. Most people will say they don't like it, that it's boring or painful, that they have no time to do it, but they're just in denial for the need to move. Well, couch potatoes, here are some more facts for you:

- In the UK, in the 16 to 24 age group, 42% failed their recommended activity level. At 65 years old, 93% of men and 96% of ladies failed too (Holford, 2009). Embarrassed, UK? You should be.
- Another study looked at 50 elderly people of an average age of 87. Given a 10 week weights workout at this age, they doubled their muscle

strength, and without any increase in walking activity, they increased their walking speed dramatically.

- In a study in Dallas, USA, five 20 year olds took to their beds for three weeks, and their readings showed a 30 year ageing effect on their aerobic activity. Then followed 8 weeks of intensive training in order to reverse the damage that occurred due to the bed rest (Saltin, 1966). These same men were revisited, as their physiology was being mapped throughout their lives. At 50, these men had gained, on average, 50 lbs in weight and had a 40% loss in cardiovascular fitness. They were then told to exercise for five out of seven days for six months, and their physiological fitness returned to that of 20 year old men.

- In a study of 1,000 people of an average age of 80, the chance of being disabled dropped 75% with an extra hour of exercise. Of the older ones, who spent 2.25 hours a week active, 25% were less likely to die. With 7 hours of exercise a week, 57% were less likely to die (Reader's Digest, 2009).

Professor Derman has hit the nail on the head here: "Exercise is the closest thing to an anti-ageing pill." There is exciting new evidence that it can increase the telomere length, our internal clock, by enhancing cell rejuvenation, so this quote is very apt indeed.

Running is an aerobic exercise known for losing dangerous belly fat, which causes inflammation and aids stress. However, there are many different aerobic exercises if running is difficult for you, including golf, sports, swimming, rowing, cross country skiing, and so on. Whatever you choose, exercise boosts your metabolic rate for up to 14 hours post exertion, helping weight and insulin as well as reducing the ageing product, glycosylated haemoglobin.

Whatever your daily aerobic exercise regime, you can be scientific about it and work with you heart rate training zone. To get this, subtract your age from 220. Then, work out 65% of this number for the lower end and 80% for the upper end of your zone. Work out in daylight whenever you can, as vitamin D is necessary to help protect you against injury. Working out helps boost your hormones, especially the human growth hormone, testosterone, and DHEA, which are all anti-ageing and immunity boosters. Your stress hormones will go down as well, slow wave sleep is boosted, and of course, it boosts bone strength – win win.

Aerobic Training

This is how you condition the heart and build aerobic stamina. Every day, I am asked, "Which aerobic exercise is best for me?" and the answer is: the one you most enjoy and will keep doing. Its nickname is cardio for a reason: like a car being driven at a faster speed, our body needs more fuel and burns it efficiently, using lots of oxygen. Your lungs take the oxygen out of the air like a giant exhaust pipe, breathing out its by-products. Your heart is a muscle that gets fitter with aerobic exercise, as the fitter you get, the less it needs to exert itself during activity. A fit dude has a strong heart with a high stroke volume, pumping more blood per beat, like having a bigger fuel tank in your car.

I noticed when I ran more that my cold hands and feet were not so bad, as my circulation was responding to training, my little arteries and capillaries having a good blow out. This keeps my blood pressure in good order, and my intercostal muscles in my rib cage respond to their new demands as my lungs show off. All the little sacs in my lungs – the alveoli – transfer oxygen better, and this is especially important to me, as I have a history of bronchitis in cold weather ever since I was a nipper. I also find that I can eat more calories as I boost my metabolic rate with aerobic exercise, so I can stay trimmer and eat a fair share of calories, and as I adore cooking and eating, this is a godsend. I am much better at recovering from an illness if I am fit, so my immune system loves it.

I also need exercise to feel more content; I tend to produce far too much adrenaline and then get an acidic stomach, but if I run this out, I reverse it all. Brain chemistry gets rejigged with more happy juice like a serotonin blast, and also soothing endorphins as well – like I feel if I give myself a bit of acupuncture or a massage, but more intense. I find my winter blues melt away and even a weaker sun gives outside exercise a lift. Also, the combo helps with sleep. I often get asked, "Should I sweat a cold out with exercise?" and the simple answer to this is no. Your immune system is fighting for you, so rest and stay away from people for the first three days – spreading germs through gyms in the winter is selfish.

Remember the heart rate check? Well, if you are very tired or emotional, check it. Above your heart rate training zone, you are training in exhaustion, anaerobically and beyond your comfort zone. I check my pulse and take a breather, walking it out until I am back in my zone. If I am feeling very tired or emotional, I am kinder to my heart. My younger, very fit brother gave me a heart monitor, and it was useful to play with in the beginning, as you soon get to know yourself with experience. For example, even the fastest pace of walking can probably leave you short of your optimum training zone by 5%, however, it's well worth exploring. I find that my running builds what I call my constant pace training – that's my aerobic endurance for general fitness. If I was to return to my tennis, I would need to do interval training, as you need to be able to stop and start quickly, using bursts of muscle activity without injury. You need to get your heart ready to cope with high surges in demand, like when you accelerate to overtake another car, and circuit training is another example of this. I always push a little throughout my exercise, although hills do this for me anyway!

Walking

Later on in this chapter, I talk about the importance of posture in walking, breathing deeply, and checking arm movements – big arm movements look clumsy. However, when the arms pump in rhythm, it's a great feeling and poles are a nice add on. Walking is a nice bum workout, ladies, so make sure you keep the pelvis even, as if your hips are headlights, and enjoy that tightening feeling in your thighs and in your bum on foot push off. Work that stomach and pelvic floor with little tightening drills, shout out positive mantras, and work out exciting, creative plans using all that helpful oxygen in the brain. Enjoy striding through and make sure your foot alignment and footwear is correct, as will be mentioned shortly. Tight calves love a stretch and weak muscles will benefit from pulling up your forefoot to avoid shin pains.

Weak ankles enjoy a wobble board workout to protect you for uneven ground. I am flat-footed myself, so my shoes support my arch, are cushioning to lessen the impact on bones, supportive to my floppy old feet, and nice and light and so comfy around my ankles. Keep altering your pace to avoid boredom, and stress your system to keep it on its toes. If you listen to music while walking, watch out for cars; I choose not to, as I run on tiny lanes with tractors and all sorts ready to flatten me, and I need to hear for safety.

I have always been more of a natural swimmer, and I love the sea and open pools; inside is a little duller and I feel like a fish in a tank without scenery. My fish tanks at home are full of underwater gardens – a bit too small for me though. I mix my running with swimming, pilates and cycling, as too much pounding on the ol' roads is not kind to our joints. I have never run a marathon – or at least not yet – mainly due to my knee. Until recently, it would swell up and ache, but then it was fixed with my magnetic resonance treatment (MRT), and there will be more about this specialist clinic in my next book. My love of the biology of cells led to me going to Germany to bring this revolutionary cell regeneration technology back to the UK, and as well as helping countless others, it has helped me too – I can now run again.

My fascination with cells, along with the lack of regeneration of cartilage in joints too old to repair, led me to Frankfurt to see the MRT time machines in action. I would add here that a dear friend – Vinod Kathuria – came out with Alan and myself to look at this research, and out of the three latest machines, one of them is with friends in Stamford, so they are all now docked in the UK. Just to say here – not only did it totally transform my fitness levels, but MRT helped Michael 'Magic Michael' van der Mark, with his broken toe bones. A real treasure to treat and he went on to repeatedly win at World Superbikes. Both he and Leon Haslam have been wonderful to meet – go for it guys! By the way, Michael's personal trainer is 80 years old!

Talking of forms of surgery, in the UK alone, six million people have arthritis, with a lot of cases made worse by lifestyle issues. Out of those who have surgery for replacement joints, 3.6% (that's 236,000), sadly die – you may have a family member who was a statistic. I remember when I was 12 writing a long essay about cloning human parts to replace bits of the body, and now I can do it in a painless, risk-free way.

Running

I am always tensing my shoulders and arms when I run, so I have to force myself to relax, and my habit of carrying a phone and keys with me doesn't 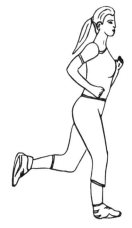 help. I love the feeling of relaxed hands, and straightening out my arms and giving them a shake often helps; I like how it strengthens my tum and back, and tightening tummy drills whilst running will also help. Then I can feel my gluts powering my leg forward, helped by my hams. I land softly on my heels, roll through my whole foot, and take off from my toes. There are so many different styles and you just need to find yours, although throwing your legs and bouncing will just wear you out and put too much weight through your knees. When I put on my winter pounds, I am careful to get my weight back to where I want it, as I know that four times my weight sits on my poor old knees.

Exercise 13 in appendix.

I also pop my ankle weights on and do some resistive weight workouts whilst writing, just to maintain muscle strength. [See appendix for exercises 7,8,12,14]. I also do pilates core workouts. [Exercises 3,29,30,39]. With the start of osteoarthritis changing with age and injury, it's a must to keep muscles strong for high impact activity in order to avoid inflammation. Treadmills bore me – it's warm inside, what else can I say? Your bum and hams are also worked less hard as roads don't have belts. I always mix fast walking with jogging and running; this is a great mix for everyone and gets beginners started injury-free. Life is about challenging yourself, so don't stop doing this with running – variety is the spice of life, after all. Run in different places, away from car fumes when possible, and make sure you keep inspired; I go through phases when I cycle more than I run, then get bored, then change.

I have a biomechanics lab at my clinic, so I can check out my biomechanics and get an orthotic adjustment as needed – more talk of this in my next book. Also, I go to running shops to check video footage of my trainers (this shows foot alignment in shoes in order to look at their suitability, which you can then add your own prescription insoles to). I wear fluorescent gear for safety and a GPS watch, thanks to my very fit younger brother, who ran with me in a relay race last summer. This is one of those events that are put on mostly for expert runners, and I sponsored our local runners, Stafford Harriers, who do some great work for kids. My brother and his friend ran like greyhounds, while myself and my colleague, David, well, what can I say… we won't be giving up the day job!

My old friend and talented shoulder surgeon turned to cycling after a lifetime of running, as he understood the importance of protecting his joints, and in recent years, ex-Olympian steeplechaser Roger turned to a lower impact sport – mind you, he hasn't had MRT yet! I remember that while on a sports medicine training course in the Canaries, I gave him pain relief treatment with acupuncture when he cut his foot on a rock in the ocean. Eastern medicine was not in his belief system, so the numbing affect puzzled the old bugger. More on treatment techniques in my next book.

Cycling

I love cycling, and I have a mountain bike equipped with amazing night lights, something which is vital, especially in the dark winter months. I got fed up with constant flats gained by riding out over nearby Cannock Chase, so that's another thing to be aware of. If you're new to cycling, first of all make sure you get your saddle in the right place: they say 10 to 15 slope to help the back, with your knees almost fully extended on the lowest point of pedal to floor. Don't get into the habit of having a sloppy back posture – it will hurt you.

Toe clips help the muscles in the back of your legs work, but just make sure they can slip off quickly in emergencies. Also make sure you wear protective clothing and use both brakes – there are many hills over somewhere like Cannock Chase, and unfortunately, coming off is very easy to do. Because of this, I take a mobile and repair kit, as I don't want my body to be found years later in a ditch! Scenery is great for the soul, just as cycling itself is great for your body. When I am avoiding dark winter nights, I will go to a spin class, attend the gym, swim, or do a pilates/yoga drill at home. If I cycle more often, I spend more time doing muscle stabilising exercises, and I find that my spin classes incorporate this really well. It's great to attend exercise classes to learn a different way of doing things, not to mention the social aspect, which can really encourage you to keep going, even when you don't feel like it.

To avoid problems with cycling, you need to address some muscle imbalance issues. Hip flexors, hams, and quads get strong, bottom muscles (the gluts) get weak, shins get tight, ankles get overused, a round shouldered position gives tight pectorals, and traps can irritate nerves in this area. Also, the lumbar spine does not like the lengthy flexed position with a stiff pelvis. I put energy into adductor – and especially abductor – leg lifts with my ankle weights, and I stretch out with the cobra [exercise 27 in appendix] to extend my lower back, before stretching my quads, hip flexors, and hams [exercises 35, 11]. Then, for your arms, add in triceps strengthening [exercise 25], corkscrew pilates movements [exercise 15], or yoga stretches – whichever you prefer.

Aerobic Gym Exercise

When I do my aerobic exercises, I like to warm up first with pre-weights, and I also tend to have a play on a cross trainer, stepper, or rower, as it's a good idea to train different muscle groups. I use the stepper to give my knees a boost, and these are particularly handy for my skier patients. The cross country skier piece of equipment is handy pre-season too, you just need a good core before using it to protect your back. The elliptical action of the cross trainer makes it a good all round exerciser, and due to its low impact, it is particularly great for injured runners.

If you need to get fit for sport, ask your gym instructor to devise a tailor-made circuit training session including skipping, boxing, shuttle runs, climbing, plyometrics, and trampolining/rebounding, which is kinder on the knees. I have a rebounder at home for a quick energy burst when writing. I will cover weights in a following section, but right now it's a quick look at core workouts to protect you from injury. Then it's all about aerobic exercise, and here we're going to take a more in-depth look at some of my favourite sports.

Essential Lumbar Stability Drill and Core Exercises

These show you how to isolate and engage the deep stabilising muscles of the pelvis and spine, the transversus abdominis, the pelvic floor, and the multifidus muscles. To get the best stability, contract the pelvic floor at the same time as pulling the tummy button in to the spine (called hollowing) in order to engage the transversus abdominis.

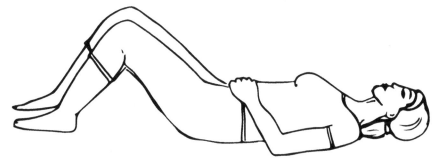

Exercise 03 in appendix.

Breathing and Stabilising Exercise

The aim here is simply to isolate and strengthen the deep postural muscles of the stomach, spine, and pelvic floor, while the brain works the diaphragm with the deep stomach muscles.

1) Get into a comfortable position on your back, with your knees bent.
2) Gently roll your hips backward and forward until you get to the neutral position for your pelvis.

3) Take a deep, slow breath into your tummy to fill up your stomach (the lower lobes of the lungs should be full of air).

4) Breathe out whilst pulling the tummy button in towards the spine, strongly at 100%. This sets the transverse abdominis.

5) Practise pulling in to a third of this, maximum – this is a nice tension to exercise to.

Pelvic Floor
Exercise 17 in appendix.

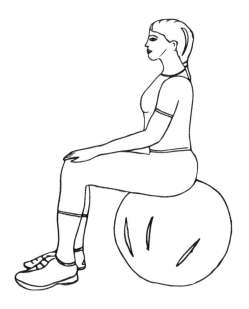

This exercise involves sitting on a fitball, or a chair if you prefer. In pilates they call this 'zipping up'.

1) When on the fitball or chair, you need to gently hollow in the tummy muscles.

2) Imagine the pelvic floor is a lift in a building, and also imagine the different floors.

3) Breathe in to fill your tummy with air, then breathe out and draw up the pelvic muscles just to floor 1.

4) Repeat for 2, then 3 – as if going up one floor at a time.

You can use these techniques as building blocks to everything.

Now we're going to look at pilates and a small selection of general back and abdominal exercises that I do at least three times a week.

Abdominals
Exercise 39 in appendix.

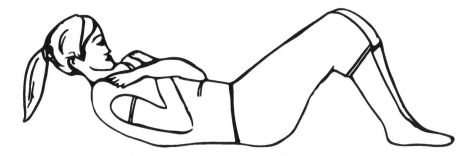

1) Lie on your back with your knees bent and your feet flat on the floor.
2) Breathe in to your stomach and then slowly breathe out, pulling in your stomach to your spine.
3) With your hands cupping your head and your chin in, lift your head a short distance and then look through your knees.
4) Hold for a few seconds and then gently go down, still holding your tummy and breathing out.
5) For a diagonal curl, lift up as before, and then this time, bring your elbow towards your opposite knee.

Spine Curl (Bridge Abs)
Exercise 28 in appendix.

1) Get into a crook lying position.
2) Lift yourself up bottom first, then imagine one vertebra at a time, until your thighs are in a straight line with the torso.

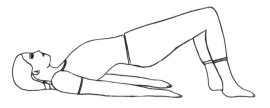

3) Lower yourself onto the floor, doing the reverse motion.

I also do this on my fitball.

Stabilisation Superman
Exercise 30 in appendix.

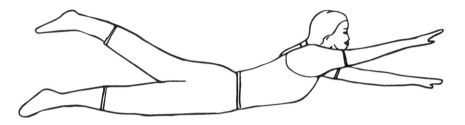

1) Lie on your tummy.
2) Set your tummy at 30%.
3) Breathe out slowly whilst lifting and lowering your opposite leg and arm.

Stabilisation Flexion
Exercise 06 in appendix.

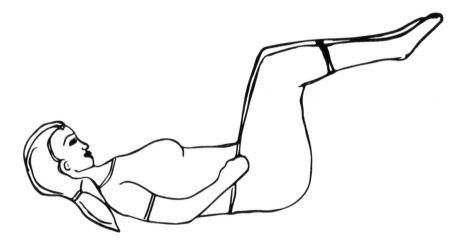

1) Activate core to 30%.
2) Lift one knee towards your chest at 90 degrees before lowering it and doing the same with the other leg. Maintain the core at all times and breathe out gently.

Stabilisation Dead Bug

Exercise 29 in appendix.

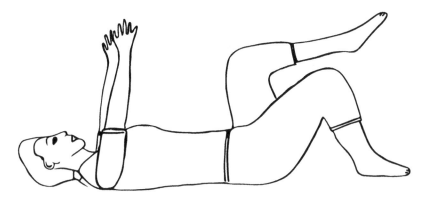

1) Take up posture of previous exercise, but this time lift your arm (the opposite one to your knee) up over your head.
2) Activate core to 30%.
3) Maintain steady tummy breathing as you open your opposite arm and leg towards the floor.
4) Return to the middle slowly.

Swimming

I love swimming. Different strokes use different muscles, and I tend to alternate my favourites: breaststroke and front crawl. I used to do sub aqua around the world and being a strong swimmer is imperative to survival. Before that, I worked as a lifeguard during my school holidays, so swimming has always been something I've been interested in.

The most important thing you have to remember is that swimming must be done in water you are safe to swim in. The sea (as well as rivers) can have strong currents and can challenge even the strongest swimmer, leaving people disorientated and fatigued – so be safe. On a personal level, I have had a few moments diving through caves and in rough seas when the tide was strong and the temperature too cold.

One day I made a big mistake in the rough sea off Devon. I had recently come back from diving in the Caribbean, and my physiology hadn't changed and my suit wasn't warm enough. I could easily have died, and I experienced headaches for weeks afterwards from coming to the surface too fast. I had trained very hard, but the weather conditions were too much for me and the team.

Anyway, back to my favourite strokes. Breaststroke demands good spinal flexibility and knee rotation and is a nice, gentle warm up stroke, whereas front crawl gets in some more powerful leg kicks from the hip to firm up the stomach. I am often asked if you can swim when you have a weak spine. On the whole, it helps if you have a strong spine, and pre-training pilates and flexibility work is needed, especially if your techniques are poor.

For the front crawl, I breathe out under water and breathe in every third stroke, alternating sides. The arms should reach out in front of you with the hands in a slightly cupped position, and then you should pull through the central line of your body with your elbow slightly flexed. A float can be used for legs or arms to alter the dynamics. I have to wear goggles so I can see without sore eyes, which is a big safety bonus – this way, I won't swim into a shark in the ocean, or hit a wall when swimming in a pool! I swim in a lovely local spa pool at Hoar Cross near my clinic, where I can meet up with friends and check on my patients and colleagues.

In the summer months, I swim in a shared pool by a beautifully renovated lighthouse and my little second home in Norfolk. I love my unspoilt wild beach and the ocean, and I am very respectful of her as she has claimed a few lives over the years. I only swim in the ocean when she is calm, running along the beach when she is rough, as well as photographing and painting her inspiring beauty and the wonderful big skies there.

When I used to do a lot of swimming – I rarely missed a day – I would make sure my pilates workouts helped with my poor upper body posture, and this is what I suggest you do if swimming is your main form of exercise. My lats (muscles in the back) were a little too strong, and my internal shoulder rotators too powerful compared to the external ones, which if not addressed, means impingement in the shoulder later in life. My shoulder blade control wasn't good enough, my pectorals were far too tight, and my neck extensors were out working my flexors. I actually still ache there. My stomach was wonderfully strong in those days, to the detriment of my back, and it could have been a lot worse if I hadn't have done my workouts and stretches.

For posture issues, there are several stretches you can focus on. For example, yoga stretches for arms are lovely, as well as:

- Pilates triceps workout – exercise 25 in appendix.
- The dumb waiter – exercise 21 in appendix.
- The corkscrew – exercise 15 in appendix.
- Stretching hip flexors will stretch out the lumbar spine with an initial rest position – exercise 35 in appendix.
- The cobra – exercise 27 in appendix.
- The child pose – exercise 10 in appendix.
- The flat superman – exercise 30 in appendix.

Injury Prevention in Tennis

I thought I would pop this in, as before I ran my own clinic, I enjoyed heading off to play tennis – now, it's a run or a swim each day, whenever a gap appears in my busy schedule. As a young child (then teenager) I played tennis every day at school, weather permitting. I remember that when I started playing, I would run over to the courts with my hard backed French books, and we would use them as rackets to practise during every morning break; the gates weren't locked, so it was my own secret tennis club. I remember Tracey (my then chum) and I would enjoy hitting tennis balls across the court with our books, dressed in normal clothes and shoes and feeling free and naughty.

Being young, I avoided injuries, but I couldn't get away with that now! This is how you can avoid too many injuries yourself:

- Make sure you play on a non-slippy court, not too cold, with good footwear and clothes and a quality racket and balls. Having well-made clothes and equipment will all reduce the chance of injury.
- Reduce the total amount of weight bearing exercises you do. Do some cross training to reduce impact loading, while still maintaining training volume.
- Light meals only, with a good fluid uptake, and make sure you are well rested pre-game.
- Mix training sessions with different activities, for example, cycling and swimming.
- If you want to be very serious about tennis – not like me with my French books – set up a training diary recording rest days, sleep, heart rate, and heart rate recovery time.

Tennis Top Tips

These tips were taught to me by my very handsome tennis coach when I was a teenager. He was so handsome, in fact, that I just had to keep playing and playing and playing…

- Practise hitting the ball in the 'sweet spot' of the racket. The shot feels good and the impact force will be at a minimum.
- Improve your stroking technique – sounds rude – especially backhand.
- Modern rackets do not absorb shock like the old ones, so to reduce the impact on your arm:
    - ◊ Lower the string tension.
    - ◊ Increase the flexibility of the racket.
    - ◊ Increase the racket head size.
    - ◊ Add lead tape to the head to increase weight.
    - ◊ Increase the grip size. The optimum grip circumference equals the   distance from the tip of the ring finger to the crease in the middle of the palm (proximal crease).
    - ◊ Grip higher up on the handle than you probably are.
    - ◊ Loosen your grip on the handle.
- Don't paint your racket – it looks crap! I only did it once as a kid.

- Play on an appropriate surface. If you play on a hard surface, the forces through the joints are much higher: twice your body weight when walking, 3 to 4 times on running and 12 times on jumping. Very dry and hard surfaces can also cause twisting ligament injuries to the knees, due to the increased friction between your shoes and the ground.
- Get a biomechanical assessment, and if you need them, purchase bespoke high quality orthotics. Make sure your footwear is appropriate.
- Train at an intensity lower than competitive, add in more relaxation time, and spend more time on cool down post activity.
- Eat healthily and adjust your calorie intake to your activity level. Take carbs for fuel, protein for rebuilding muscle, high quality vitamin and mineral supplements, and make sure you drink plenty of water.
- Enjoy the stress relief that exercise can bring and don't force yourself if you are exhausted, as this is when you are most likely to get injured.
- Get regular sports massages to remove trouble spots before they become injuries.

Warming Up and Cooling Down

Warming up is often overlooked and should be part of your injury prevention routine, as there are a number of benefits:

- The muscles work better when warm and oxygenated with good blood flow.
- The joints become more flexible which reduces the pull on the muscles.
- The nervous system becomes more responsive.

Including a gentle jog in your warm up will give the muscles the energy supply they need to work properly. Follow this with sport specific exercises and dynamic, sport specific stretching drills – this regime has largely replaced old fashioned static alternatives. Examples of tennis specific exercises are running for 5 to 20 minutes with your heels up to your buttocks, or with high knees up to the hip level. Increasing the size and speed of movements – as the body warms up and the heart rate increases – will more closely simulate competitive conditions. It is also important to focus on full body conditioning, as predominantly one sided sports – such as tennis – can cause muscle imbalances.

You should allow a total exercise and stretch time of 15 to 30 minutes and no more than 30 minutes before competing, otherwise the benefits will be lost. Cool down should include a gentle jog plus light stretching to help eliminate waste products (the polite words for it) and reduce muscle soreness.

Pilates for Tennis

These include:

- Abdominal drill – exercises 3 and 6 in appendix.
- Shoulder stretches, the dumb waiter – exercise 21 in appendix.
- The corkscrew – exercise 15 in appendix.
- Spine curls – exercise 5 in appendix.
- Hams stretch – exercise 11 in appendix.
- Hip flexors and quads stretch – exercise 35 in appendix.

Football

With so many people playing football, injuries during training and matches are commonplace. Even the fittest and best prepared are not immune: the 2002 World Cup saw a total of 171 injuries from 64 matches, equivalent to 2.7 injuries per match. Of these, over half the injuries resulted in the player missing training or a match. Even the physios who look after you get injured – poor Gary Lewin broke his ankle recently when England was playing away in Brazil. I was impressed with what a kind, caring gentleman he is and he also makes good tea – very important.

So, what causes football injuries?

- Player age: older players have generally sustained previous injuries and are more susceptible to the injury reoccurring.
- Body preparation: poor fitness, weak muscles, or inappropriate training can all lead to injury.
- Inadequate game preparation and overexertion: inadequate warm up can lead to strains and sprains.
- Pitch condition: poor pitches increase the risk of sprained ankles and knees.
- Equipment: incorrect footwear can lead to foot or ankle injuries and can eventually lead to chronic problems in the ankle, knee, hip, and lower back.
- Contact injuries, including fighting: cuts, grazes, ligament/tendon damage, and even fractures can be the result of contact injuries.
- Tiredness: can lead to mistimed tackles, and poor balance and coordination.

The greatest type of injury cause has been shown to be previous injuries, and this is a major factor particularly in hamstring and groin muscle strains, as well as knee and ankle ligament sprains. Without the correct rehabilitation and treatment programme, there is a much greater risk of the injury reoccurring.

Common Football Injuries

By far the most common football injuries are muscle strains and ligament strains. My football physio told me of a recent study that looked at injuries in the top 50 European football clubs, and it was reported that the single most common injury subtype was thigh strain, accounting for 17% of all injuries over a number of seasons. Traumatic injuries, such as fractures or complete ruptures, were more common during the competitive season – need I say more!

So here's my suggestion of a pilates drill for you, although I don't play football so I won't be joining you on this one.

Pilates Drill

- Core abdominal drills – exercises 3, 6 and 39 in appendix.
- Spine curl – exercise 5 in appendix.
- Yoga curl down – exercise 42 in appendix.
- Hams stretches – exercise 11 in appendix.
- Quads and hip flexor stretches – exercise 35 in appendix.

Why Do I Need A Strong Core?

Why do you need a strong core? Well, here is a fine example involving a well-known sportsman, and I shall call this delightful international football player 'Sam'. I was asked one late, snowy evening to head out to a hotel close to a football stadium the night before an important match. Sam was very fearful about playing, as he was plagued by hamstring injuries, as well as some more imaginary injuries.

Sam was amazing at scoring goals, but not so much recently. Assessment showed me a link with his spine, referring pain into his hams. I sorted out the spinal problem and then explained to his physiotherapist and coach that his rehab programme had to be changed in order to divert a lot more attention to core work. This would protect his spine as the postural curves were far from ideal and the shape had become fixed over time. Every training session directed Sam's attention to his core, and he started to score again. So you see, you can be an Olympic athlete or a football star, but an insidious injury can still fool your body's muscles into not protecting you properly.

Horse Riding

Due to where I live and work, nearly all of my patients have horses, and my late grandpa was a bit of a horse whisper, so he would have loved that. Getting the best out of riding needs both the rider and the horse to be fit and prepared. Unfortunately, riders tend to put themselves second, and don't realise how much this impacts their enjoyment and performance. So, it is important that your therapist cares for you – the rider – as much as you care for your horse. I see a lot of avoidable spinal, shoulder, and hip pain, so just take a moment to write down the activities you do and look for clues to your problem:

- Lifting heavy water pails or hay bales.
- Mucking out.
- Poor posture.
- Lack of fitness, core strength, and flexibility, leading to poor saddle balance.
- Rigid joints or weak muscles.

Any biomechanical abnormalities will cause you to ride unevenly and this will reflect in your horse because the horse feels your every movement. Your motor skills and body control adjusts the horse's muscles, and with time, poor saddle balance will lead to your horse injuring itself and possibly you as well. Conditions such as an arthritic hip or poor spinal control will reflect in timing and these imperfections get mirrored in the horse's musculature.

Whatever your injury, I encourage you to have good core stability and correct any biomechanical imbalances before returning to riding. Here are a few preventative tips:

- When injured, treat yourself to box rest and get assessment and treatment.
- On cold days, warm up first – groom the horse and stretch out.
- Cool off and stretch out afterwards, quickly replacing clothing.
- See a personal fitness instructor about core strength, flexibility, and stamina.
- Eat healthily to promote joint flexibility.
- Wear the correct safety gear.

Over the years, I have helped patients and friends with rounded shoulders, over tight hip flexors, tight adductors, stretched achilles, poor shoulder blade control, weak tummy muscles, and strained back muscles. I remember one Olympian athlete who I treated – they had a totally destroyed hip joint but still bravely rode through the pain.

There are some great pilates exercises that sort all this out, if done regularly:

- Stretching the spine out with spine curls – exercise 42 in appendix.
- The resting forward stretch – exercise 10 in appendix.
- Adductor – exercise 2 in appendix.
- Hip flexor and quads stretches – exercise 35 in appendix – are essential.
- If doing my leg weight exercises, I avoid adductor.
- Stomach curls are useful – exercise 39 in appendix.
- Shoulder posture corrections such as the dumb waiter (exercise 21 in appendix) and the corkscrew (exercise 15 in appendix).
- Yoga shoulder stretches in sitting position – exercise 37 in appendix.

May I just add to this section that the action of horse riding is generally nice for the spine. I remember when a previous patient and friend, Doug, bought a mechanical horse to the hospital – it was something he and Princess Anne were working on to do with the kids riding for the disabled, and the rider was attached to a computer to show the pelvic movements. It was great fun and it proved a point about keeping your spine mobile, as long as you stay on the horse!

Hockey

The demands of training and playing – from club matches to the England squad – week on week constantly pushes your body to the limit, so remaining in optimum health is imperative as a hockey player, and the adage "prevention is better than cure" has never been more pertinent, as the demands placed on the body get greater and for longer periods. You can't get 'spare parts' for your body, so it's important to do everything you can to prevent injuries.

There are two main causes of injury in hockey:

- <u>Direct</u>: usually as a result of a fall or blow, e.g. cuts, astro turf burn, dislocations, breaks, or impact injuries.
- <u>Indirect</u>: muscular injuries can occur as a result of overuse, not warming up or cooling down correctly, or from being under recovery.

It is very likely that every player will sustain at least some type of injury during their playing career. Some of these injuries may be so severe that they demand hospital treatment, but most hockey injuries involve damage to the soft tissues and will be best helped by a physiotherapist.

Injury statistics from English Hockey's elite squads identifies that the majority of injuries are biomechanical in nature, rather than being due to acute trauma, although personally, I have recently looked after a lot of patients with head trauma, either due to falling on their head or being hit by the ball.

Common Hockey Injuries

Common hockey injuries include:

- Sprained ankles.
- Hamstring strains.
- Groin strains.
- Knee cartilage injuries.
- Lower back pain.
- Cruciate ligament injuries.
- Facial injuries.
- Contusions – muscular damage and bleeding caused by contact with the ball or stick.

Injury Prevention

Here are several things you can do to prevent the above injuries from occurring when playing hockey:

- <u>Warm up and cool down</u>: these should be performed before and after matches and training to prepare your body for activity and to return it to a state of rest afterwards.
- <u>Core stability</u>: this is essential to both performance and injury prevention; if you have a weak core, you cannot build strong movements or forces on top of it [exercises in appendix 3, 617, 39].
- <u>Biomechanical assessment</u>: this is to assess for leg length discrepancy, foot posture, muscle length, and strength differences, which may cause or lead to injury. Many of these differences can be corrected with orthotics, as well as stretching or strengthening exercises. A very high percentage of injuries in hockey are from overuse or due to poor core stability and biomechanics.
- <u>Sports massage</u>: this is to keep muscles relaxed, lactate free, and in optimum condition for optimum performance.

Top tip: listen to your body. Niggles are a warning sign that there is a problem!

Cricket

Whilst thinking about touching on cricket, I found an old newspaper cutting on my late Uncle Cyril. He lived for cricket, and he was the chairman of Warwickshire. He even had a suite named after him, and I asked him if it was the toilet block! He was a wicket keeper for England, and he helped raise funds for the first angiogram. Anyway, wicket keepers are in an uncomfortable position of squatting behind stumps, with their head back and arm out – poor old back and fingers. Uncle Cyril broke a few.

Anyway, a lot of my professional cricketers hurt their lower back, especially fast bowlers, who tend to suffer from either a condition called spondylolisthesis or stress fracture. West Indians don't tend to suffer as much, as they're more bendy. Fielders, with their twisting motion throws, also get achey backs, and the repetitive rotate, flex, and extend actions need good preventative stretching and strengthening exercises.

Pilates is needed to improve pelvic stability and lumbar spine stability (for these, see exercises 3, 17, 6, and 39 in appendix), as well as scapula stability (see the dumb waiter and the corkscrew, exercises 21 and 15 in appendix).

Skiing

Whilst visiting a pain clinic in Vancouver to do my instructor training, I had a day in the beautiful whistler mountains with my rather competitive colleagues. It was just like Bridget Jones – skiing down slopes on my bum was my clumsy style. My colleagues were Norwegian ski instructors, not to mention Mike and Steve, who were both ex-army physios, who found it great fun to watch my 'creative' skiing. In fact, a French ski guide once said – during a previous trip with a bunch of medics – that I 'ski like a crumpled newspaper'. We were all highly competitive, and as well as being hopeless at speed, to my embarrassment I fell out of a ski lift into a snow drift!

Anyway, in my clinical role, knees always take a hammering in skiing and I often had French clinical reports describing holiday traumas. So, if you are planning to ski, do this before you go:

- Train your quads and bum.
- Get a really strong tummy.
- Good scapula control helps with pole coordination.
- Flex your foot muscles and ankles to sustain lengthy times in boots.
- Practise good balance – a fitball is helpful here.
- Check life insurance!
- Check eyewear such as glasses, as instructors are very handsome.

For pre-skiing, try the following exercises to get ready:

- Shoulder stretches and stability – exercises 21 and 15 in appendix.
- Spine curls – exercise 5 in appendix.
- Abdominal workout – exercises 6, 3 and 39 in appendix.
- Leg stretches – exercises 11, 2, 35 and 34 in appendix.
- Leg weights for all leg muscle – exercises 12, 14, 7, and 8 in appendix.

Golf

I went off golf when a player broke my nose with a golf club at the age of nine. Back then, I thought it was very exciting because I was the centre of attention in a big drama – people were passing out as I was bleeding furiously and it didn't hurt a bit. Well, not until the tetanus bum injection, that is… then I decided that golf wasn't for me.

Many years later, in my Rowley Hall Hospital physio manager days, I was asked to do a presentation on golf and back pain, so I took myself off for lessons, and learnt that it was bloody complicated. Because of this, I decided to leave golf until retirement. However, the golf swing fascinated me and resulted in me getting robotic spinal mobile machines for my clinic (more on this in my next book). Golf is asymmetrical, repeatedly twisting the body in the same way and bending over the ball. Using the same muscles and reinforcing the same bent over posture again and again can lead to a very poor back; some muscles are repeatedly overused while others remain underused.

The golf pros and professional golfers I have treated over the years have overuse injuries in their shoulders, neck, hips, and feet, and I've read MRI evidence that shows more wear on the right side of lumbar discs and facets, for right-handed golfers. A sports massage is yummy for tight, dominating back muscles and tight pectorals – I was so tender after every lesson. I can vouch for forearms getting sore and neck extensors being overworked, and weak post scapular muscles only enhanced the round shouldered-ness and curved thoracic spine. At my first golf talk, I got my very fit muscular little brother to demo a warm up and cool down drill (I hope my older brother isn't offended!). The doctors I presented to were sitting quietly with their hands on their little pot bellies, saying that it didn't matter – they warmed up by the end of the game!

Here are some pilates and yoga warm up exercises you can use before playing golf:

- The corkscrew – exercise 15 in appendix.
- The dumb waiter – exercise 21 in appendix.
- Triceps – exercise 25 in appendix.
- Abdominal drills – exercises 3, 6, 29, and 39 in appendix.
- Spine roll downs – exercise 42 in appendix.
- Golf club behind head (pole raises) and twists.

For post-game, try:

- Spine roll downs – exercise 42 in appendix.
- Spine curls – exercise 5 in appendix.
- Abdominal drills – exercises 3, 6, and 39 in appendix.
- Back rotations – exercise 38 in appendix.
- Knee hugs – exercise 5 in appendix.
- Hip flexors/quads – exercise 35 in appendix.
- Adductors – exercise 2 in appendix.
- Hams stretches – exercise 11 in appendix.
- The cobra – exercise 27 in appendix.

Dance

I was a very young, flat-footed ballerina, but I enjoyed dressing up in the clothes, and while I don't dance anymore, the importance of balance and pose have stayed with me. The dancers I have looked after have very worn toes, feet, and knees, not to mention other knee problems and slipped discs.

I enjoyed great dancing events, doing everything from ceroc to jive. I would often dance, then pause to treat someone on the dance floor, then dance again. Main problems for dancers are overstretched muscles, ankle and foot injuries from dancing on point, tight achilles, stress fractures, overstretched knees, arthritis of the hips, and interestingly, proprioception not being good enough (proprioception is the ability of joints to know where they are in space, and is necessary for balance).

Many dancers are under pressure to carry on with the show, even after injury, and pilates can be used to centre movement, while maintaining the core helps with the imbalance of limbs. Keeping too slim can lead to osteoporosis and bone fractures.

Exercises for dancers can include:

- Abdominal workout – exercises 3, 6, and 39 in appendix.
- The cobra – exercise 27 in appendix.
- Rest position – exercise 10 in appendix.
- Arm weights and stretches – exercises 31, 32, and 33 in appendix.
- Yoga for upper limbs – exercise 37 in appendix.
- Tai chi – exercise 23 in appendix.

Actors

Those I have worked with do a lot of posture work and core work, and they stand up so smoothly at interviews, like a youngster getting out of a chair. Sex looks better with a lean, coordinated body, and remember that in amateur acting, you need to study the posture and act the age of the character you're portraying – think about how the joints move at that age, as well as the coordination and speed of the character.

Favourite exercises for actors include:

- Posture in standing, walking, and running.
- Core with lots of slow breathing work – exercise 3 in appendix.
- Abdominals – exercises 6 and 39 in appendix.
- Rest position – exercise 10 in appendix.
- Roll down – exercise 42 in appendix.
- Side rolls – exercise 38 in appendix.
- The cobra – exercise 27 in appendix.
- The corkscrew – exercise 15 in appendix.
- Tai chi, especially for the arms – exercise 23 in appendix.
- Yoga arm stretches – exercise 37 in appendix.

Musicians and Singers

Musicians – and singers in particular – need a strong neck and excellent breathing techniques. One time, I was out diving in the Caymans when I came across a handsome singer with a cricked neck, let's call him Mr Barefoot Man. I was strolling along with him and fell into a hot tub while fully dressed in a summer evening dress. I didn't even see it, and I can still remember feeling very uncool about it. A little manipulation of his neck and he was fine. Singing and playing guitar is a very asymmetrical activity for the neck, as well as the thoracic spine and shoulder girdle.

Favourite exercises for musicians and singers include:

- Breathing exercises – exercise 3 in appendix.
- Abdominal workout – exercises 6, 16, 17, 30, and 39 in appendix.
- Spine curls – exercise 5 in appendix.
- The cobra – exercise 27 in appendix.
- Rest position – exercise 10 in appendix.
- The dumb waiter (scapula control) – exercise 21 in appendix.
- The corkscrew – exercise 15 in appendix.
- Yoga for upper limbs and spine – exercise 37 in appendix.
- Finger exercises for musicians.

Fishing

Fishing really isn't my thing – it's too slow and I like swimming with fish without a hook in their mouth. However, I have treated a lot of injuries associated with casting a line using various poor techniques, causing neck, shoulder, and elbow strains. Pilates and yoga pre and post fishing sessions will help avoid injuries, and these exercises include:

- Abdominals – exercises 3 and 39 in appendix.
- Spine curls/yoga roll down – exercise 42 in appendix.
- Side rolls – exercise 38 in appendix.
- The cobra – exercise 27 in appendix.
- Rest position – exercise 10 in appendix.
- Yoga shoulder workout – exercise 37 in appendix.
- The corkscrew – exercise 15 in appendix.
- Triceps for strengthening – exercise 25 in appendix.
- Biceps strengthening – exercise 32 in appendix.

Sailing

I tried this 'hanging my bum out over the sea on a winch' thing – very hair-raising and sailing on bumpy oceans just makes me throw up; on my many diving adventures, I had to refrain from eating and take anti-sickness tablets to make sure this didn't happen. Canoeing didn't make me feel sick, it just worried me about what I might capsize into. I went on a short, fast water ride with my brother once, and he was screaming so loudly that I thought he must be extremely excited. That was, until I opened my eyes and realised my right foot was stamping on his nuts as he'd slipped across the dingy...

Sailors are prone to hunched over postures, poor shoulder posture, crushed nuts, and overuse injuries. Poor posture makes the shoulder blades stick out, traps muscles get tight, and hip flexors and upper abs get dominant. I will just add that rowers also get knee problems, with their kneecaps tracking out.

Exercises for sailors include:

- Spine stretches, forward bend – exercise 42 in appendix.
- Rest position – exercise 10 in appendix.
- The cobra – exercise 27 in appendix.
- Hip flexor and quads stretches – exercise 35 in appendix.
- Scapula workout, the corkscrew – exercise 15 in appendix.
- The dumb waiter – exercise 21 in appendix.
- Triceps – exercise 25 in appendix.
- All arm exercises with either a light weight or no weight, exercise 31 for pecs, exercise 32 for biceps.
- Yoga for posture and to open up the chest – exercise 37 in appendix.

Water-skiing

Falling from water skis injures the spinal discs, and beginners pull on the bar too much, getting round shoulders, tight pecs, shoulder impingements, and elbow strains. Exercises include:

- Abdominal drill – exercises 3 and 39 in appendix.
- Advanced stability workout – exercises 16 and 30 in appendix.
- Curl down – exercise 42 in appendix.
- Rest position – exercise 10 in appendix.
- The cobra – exercise 27 in appendix.
- Dumb waiter for shoulder/scapula posture – exercise 21 in appendix.
- Quads and hip flexor stretches – exercise 35 in appendix.
- Usual spine stretches.

Athletics

There are far too many to go through in this book, as it would be a big book in itself – javelin, discus… every track and field event has its own special issues. With steeple chasers, my only experience was treating Roger Hackney, ex Olympian, shoulder surgeon and friend, whose calves played up, and he was a stickler for very aggressive core strength and lower limb stretches.

I've tried my hand at trampolining and gymnastics, and what can I say? A double twist and pike thing went very wrong! I must admit that my brief interest in believing I could do this was due to a very handsome instructor, and I soon gave up. The gymnast and trampolining kids I went to watch in China were crazily flexible, poor little things. Athletic kick boxing classes are great for your core and for stretching, which is essential for athletes. I would just say, in general, focus on lots of strong, diaphragmatic breathing, good spinal flexibility, core work, and leg stretches. With throwing events, arm stretches and scapula stability are vitally important.

Here are some essential exercises for athletes:

- Throwers: the corkscrew and the dumb waiter, exercises 15 and 21 in appendix.
- Track events: hip and quad stretch (exercise 35 in appendix), calf (warrior, exercise 41), hams stretch (exercise 11), adductor/butterfly stretch (exercise 2), rest position (exercise 10), and abdominals (exercises 3 and 39 in appendix).
- Trampolining and gymnastics: many forms of stretches combined with core work to help stabilise overstretched joints.

Rugby

Treating these guys is tough on the old hands, and I have seen many whiplashes, groin strains, blown lumbar discs, broken bones, and torn shoulder tendons in my time. They come in with tight traps, a poor core, tight adductors, weak gluts, tight hip flexors, and worn out hams. Prop forwards get neck and shoulder issues, while wingers get tackled by heavy, fast moving humans. The semi crouch posture also irritates their backs, so many rugby players find their way to my clinic. Rehab needs alternating movement patterns, different types of exercise, and lots of stretching tight muscles. I remember when I used to visit Roger's orthopaedic office; on one occasion, he stripped off a rugby player stark bollock naked to address a groin injury and wanted me to stare professionally at his groin area… those were the days. There will be more about sorting our groins out in *The Human Garage*.

Exercises for rugby players include:

- Spine curls – exercise 5 in appendix.
- Roll downs – exercise 42 in appendix.
- Hip flexors – exercise 35 in appendix.
- Hams stretches – exercise 11 in appendix.
- Abdominal curls – exercise 39 in appendix.
- Corkscrew – exercise 15 in appendix.
- Dumb waiter – exercise 21 in appendix.

Why You Need To Use Weights

Why isn't it enough just to do aerobic exercise? Why should we go to the gym or use weights at home? Why do you need to get some muscle? First, let's look at some sobering facts:

- In the mid 80s, biochemists established that muscles are essential to immunity, as glutamine is manufactured by muscles and is key to the immune system.
- American females, aged between 20 and 80 years old, lose on average 8 lbs of healthy muscle over the years and gain 23 lbs of excess fat.
- American men, aged between 20 and 80 years old, lose a quarter of their muscle mass, and a lot of their immunity to diseases follows this.

Ladies, do you want to lose more fat and look younger? In a ten week study by Neil McCartney, it was shown that resistive exercise is part of the answer. In this study, inactive females were found to have an average of 21.8% fat (McCartney, cited in Colgan, 2005). Some of these ladies were advised to follow an aerobic exercise regime, and their fat was reduced to an average of 16.2%. Others were advised to do resistive work with weights, and they measured in at 14.7% – get my drift?

All sorts of interesting studies went on to show that resistive exercise boosts human growth hormone, testosterone, and DHEA, which are all anti-ageing and immunity boosters. Furthermore, when this happens, the stress hormone goes down, slow wave sleep is boosted, and so is bone strength. A University of Pittsburgh study looked at 2,300 people over five years and found that those with low quads strength were 51% more likely to die. A second study looked at both age and quads strength, and they found that you were 13 times more likely to die with weak quads. That should put the fear of God into you weak kneed individuals.

Here's a starting point for all you beginners out there who want to try weight training. My brother Jez used to keep his body building stuff in my garage many moons ago when he was an instructor whilst studying at university, and he taught me the basics long before I was a physio.

The limit time for resistive exercise is a max of 45 to 60 minutes in any one session, and if you have a busy day, even doing several sessions in 15 minute blocks will add up and make all the difference. You need to work different muscles with difference exercises, and even with the same muscles, you need to vary the intensity and the type of exercise in order to constantly challenge your muscles. One way of doing this is to write down a list and put them in a jar. You can then randomly pull out different ones to stop boredom from creeping in – something that my personal fitness coach at the clinic suggests doing. I would add to this that I'd like you to group lower limb, back/stomach, and upper limb exercises in order to allow the necessary recovery for your muscles to repair themselves.

Good strengthening comes from including eccentric loading (which is the muscle fibres lengthening), but make sure you never overstrain; inflammation isn't good. Muscles take five to eight days to repair and strengthen, then they start noticeably weakening without any further exercise. I teach my patients very specific exercises for their specific injuries, however, here is a starting point: start by doing an aerobic action, either by using a light weight with 8 to 12 reps, or just a warm up exercise, then work the chosen muscle with a stronger 8 to 10 repetition, pushing yourself to near exhaustion by the last one. To work a selected group of muscles, leave a minimum of 48 hours in between for healing, and take a protein drink an hour after a hard workout. Before a workout, take some glucose and hydrate well – drinking ionised water is even better – and keep an alkaline diet, as muscle work will enhance an acidic environment.

Muscles have two types of fibre: the fast and slow twitch, the former working hard during aerobic activity, and the latter in explosive actions and weight training. Unlike the constant supply of energy generated during aerobic exercise, the fast twitch can only grab energy in the muscle, hence short bursts of exertion only, before its short battery life is effectively over.

It's interesting to see so many different body shapes in my gym. There are three basic types: thin, fat and muscly was my way of remembering them at uni. Ectomorphs are those irritating friends who eat everything and stay looking slim in clothes, as it is more difficult for them to build muscle. Endomorphs are heavier; they put weight on more easily and have to diet. They can build muscle, but it is often buried under the fat, making them look bigger. Aerobic workouts are also essential here – that or big pants! Mesomorphs, on the other hand, have an athletic build, narrow waist, and broad shoulders. They build muscle easily, although they have to diet as well.

Patients ask me how heavy, how often, and how long for, and the key here is to follow a guided programme of specific coordinated exercise. I was very good at being inaccurate with my weights workout – as I got easily distracted – and once put straight and sworn at, I felt the difference of correct movement: the muscles strengthened faster with less weight. I am also asked about lifting at work; if you are trained to regularly lift a certain weight and you are strong, the risk of injury is significantly less.

Patients often ask me how much weight they should use at the gym. I found that my maximum dumbbell weight for toning was to do between

12 and 15 reps comfortably then go hard with the last 3. Then, I had to take a break before the next set. When you want to bulk up a muscle, it's the handful of hard reps that do the breaking down and rebuilding action – not particularly kind to your body. Needing to continue that feeling of toning to get gently stronger means that you have to gently increase the weight, which is a rewarding and positive thing to do. Toning means high reps of 15 or more, low exertion and only 30 seconds are needed between sets. When defining, you need to make more of an effort to do 10 to 14 reps before muscle fatigue, with only a minute to recover, then repeat. Building and stressing muscles means fatigue at a max of 10, pushing into pain for an extra couple of reps, and a minute or two's rest is essential. After injury, the first set is the first to be attempted. Pushing your strength – rather than toning – means using a weight that you can just move a maximum of 4 to 8 reps, then resting a minute or two minutes per set. The latter will lead to muscle soreness, repair, and bulking.

Free weights involve more body control and are, on the whole, more effective. I tend to work opposing or different muscles to fill the rest of the time in with an exercise for a different muscle, and it also allows more recovery time, as I don't want muscle soreness if I'm working on patients or teaching pain relieving techniques involving fine motor control. I like to teach weight work with pilates overtones to protect the back, and just to reiterate: weights are great for strengthening bones. Look at my pilates drill before using weights.

Here are some of my favourite dumbbell and Theraband exercises (you can use Theraband instead of dumbbells, especially when travelling). These exercises focus on your core.

Triceps with Pilates

Exercise 25 in appendix.

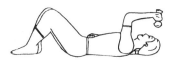 Here's one exercise that protects the neck. I have dumbbells in my office at home and I lie on a rug with music on and candles lit, then relax into a mini workout in a good posture. They're great for breaking up long sessions at your desk.

- Lie on your back, with your knees bent and your pelvis in neutral.
- Place a small cushion under your head.
- Hold the weights in your hands, above your eyes, with your arms bent at the elbow.
- Breathe in.
- Zip up, gently pull your tummy button to your spine, and push the weights up.
- Do, say, three sets of 15, or at least 12 comfortably.
- Check that your shoulder blades are softly centred towards your spine.

Biceps Curl

Exercise 1 and 32 in appendix.

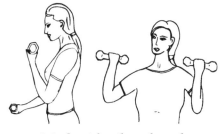

- Exercise 1, one arm at a time; Exercise 32, both arms at same time.
- Sit on a chair or fitball or stand.
- Keep back straight and still
- Gently position shoulder blades in correct posture

- Work with pilates breathe
- Hold dumbells in hands with palm downwards
- As you bend elbows turn palm upwards
- At end of movement gently straighten elbows to return
- If sitting, make sure the weight is even through your buttocks.
- Place your elbows at 90 degrees with your palms facing upwards.

- Keep your neck relaxed and stop your lower back from moving with the weights.
- Breathe in and prepare.
- As you raise one arm, breathe out and hollow your tummy.
- When your hand ends close to your shoulder, breathe in again as you extend your elbow.
- Alternate hands, or do first one arm then the next.
- Don't do any crazy rocking that I often see in the gym.
- Try 15 reps – the last 3 will be tough.
- Then increase the weight if the last 3 become easy.

I prefer you to do this exercise standing, as long as your balance is reasonable.

Pec Fly and Overhead Strokes
Exercise 31 in appendix.

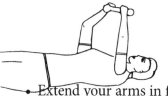

- Use the same position you did for triceps.
- Lying on your back, bend your knees.
- You can add a ball between your legs to squeeze.
- Extend your arms in front of your chest, with your elbows just a little off straight.
- With the breathing, one example is to breathe in as you bring your arms up and out on a downward movement.
- Gently hollow your tummy as usual with breathing.

I like to alter this exercise and take both arms up over my head together, then alternate it as if swimming backstroke.

Strengthening Hams
Exercise 7 in appendix.

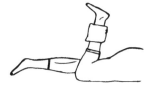

- Lie on stomach and place weight on your ankle
- Begin with knee straight and slowly bend knee towards bottom with knee steady
- Return leg and repeat

Strengthening Quads

Exercise 8 in appendix.

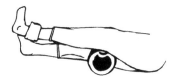

- Place weight on ankle of involved leg and put a rolled up towel under knee, or sit on fitball.
- Lift leg and lock out knee
- Slowly lower down

Lateral Rotator, Rotator Cuff

Exercise 33 in appendix.

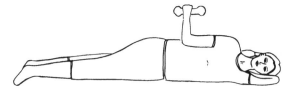

The lateral rotator works a shoulder muscle called the infraspinatus and protects the shoulder function to minimise changes of impingement with posture and age issues. This one I combine with my adductor/abductor hip strengthening leg exercises, using my ankle weights.

- Lie on your side and strap the ankle weights on your ankles.
- Keep a neutral position of your pelvis.
- Stretch out your lower arm and pop a towel under your ear for comfort.
- Have your knees bent a little.
- Gently hollow your tummy by breathing in the usual way.
- To work your infraspinatus muscle, keep your elbow at 90 degrees with the dumbbell, and gently rotate your hand out with your elbow held to your side.
- Do three sets of 12.
- Alternate sides then start hip work.

Exercise 12 in appendix.

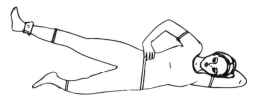

For this, do the above, then:
- Have your upper knee about six inches above the floor.

- Straighten out your knee, flex your ankle and turn your toes down slightly.
- Lift upper leg another six inches as you breathe out and pull in button to protect your back.
- Breathe in as you lower and repeat about a dozen times before putting your leg down and turning over.

Exercise 14 in appendix.

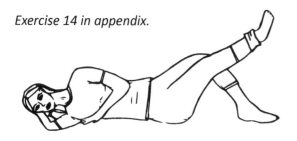

- Now bend your upper leg and stretch out your lower leg.
- Push the top leg in front of the body and rest it.

- Hollow and contract your   pelvic floor, breathing in as you lower to protect your back.
- Lift your lower leg up – with ankle weights on – and move gently up and down to six inches above the floor for 12 to 20 times maximum.
- You can stretch it out in this position.

Flexibility

I am finding that as I age, I am stiffer and less flexible, as age brings with it less elastic joints. Regular stretching is now essential to make me feel fluid and comfortable, and I know that it's helping my joints as well. I like sitting on a fitball, which helps to prevent the shortening of hip flexors and hams and which lessens the curve in your back stressing discs. Some people have hypermobility and must not overstretch, and pregnant mums also have ligament laxity. Stretching before exercise is much less important than after exercise, when muscles are warm. Ten minutes a day is good preventative care for your body.

We have physiotherapy guidelines for flexibility norms, which means the normal amount of movement in a joint. If your joints are stiff, it can be a sign of early osteoarthritis, or an injury. If too flexible, you need to avoid activities that overstretch and get a good pilates regime going.

- Neck rotation: turning right to left, look at the midline to turn your head. Less than 75 degrees is poor, 75 to 85 is normal, and above 85 degrees is too flexible.
- Shoulders: up to 170 degrees elevation is poor, showing stiffness, and above 180 degrees is too flexible.
- Straight leg raise: lift it into the air. Up to 75 degrees is poor hamstring flexibility, over 90 degrees is too much flexibility.
- Quads: up to 130 degrees is poor, over 150 degrees is too much.

Western Stretches

These are some of my favourite 'Western' stretches. Many of them are similar to yoga stretches, however, and are often interchangeable.

Neck
Exercise 43 in appendix.

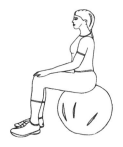

I like to do mine on the fitball.

- Tilt your ear to one side and then the other.
- With your head in a neutral position, turn first to the right then the left.

The Corkscrew
Exercise 15 in appendix.

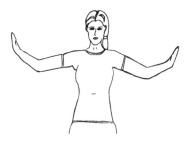

- Breathe out and prepare your core.
- Float your arms up and out and place your hands behind your head.
- Breathe in as you shrug your shoulders to your ears.
- Breathe out as you drop them down.
- Breathe in as you bring your elbows back a little and your shoulder blades get closer together.
- Breathe out as your arms come down to the side.

151

Dumb Waiter

Exercise 21 in appendix.

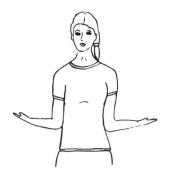

- Stand or sit.
- Prepare your core.
- Have your elbows tucked in and your palms facing up.
- Take your hands back, opening them and keeping your shoulder blades down.
- Breathe out and return to start.

Back stretches and spine curls are also good exercises.

Rest Position

Exercise 10 in appendix.

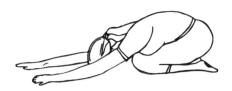

Don't do this exercise if you have a sore back.

- Get into the rest position.
- Come up onto all fours.
- Keep your arms still and sit back onto your feet.
- Breathe pilates style.
- Placing your legs further apart gives the chest a deeper stretch.

Spinal Roll Down

Exercise 42 in appendix.

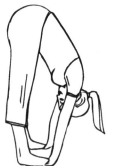

This has been previously explained, but gently lean down from standing and come up slowly, unrolling.

Knee Rolls

Exercise 38 in appendix.

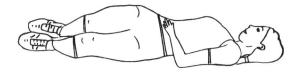

- Lie on your back with your knees together and your feet on the floor.
- Do a pilates breath.
- Roll your knees from one side to the other.

Knee Hug

Exercise 5 in appendix.

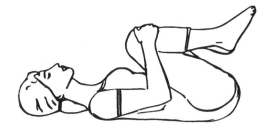

For this, simply lie on your back and hug your knees. if you find a double knee bend too difficult bend in one knee at a time (exercise 9 in appendix).

Other popular stretches include the child pose, the forward flex, the cobra, the cat/dog yoga pose, the butterfly, and abduction without using ankle weights. See the yoga section for more on these.

Quads Stretch, Side Lie

Exercise 35 in appendix.

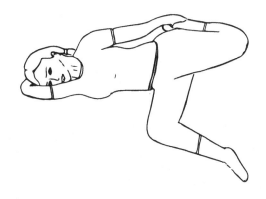

Quads run along the front of the thigh and flex the knee and hip. The hip flexors run along here too. I tend to put a hand on a wall to steady me, breathe in and out, hollow and zip and bend a foot towards my bottom, then breathe normally for at least 20 seconds. I tend to do this after a run when nice and warm. For hams stretch, start with an adductor stretch, while sitting. Sit with your knees bent and with the soles of your feet together, then gently stretch out your knees in a butterfly-like posture and hold for 20 to 30 seconds. Then, practise gentle tummy hollowing. For quads side lie and hip flexor exercises, assume the position I use for side lying: bend your knees to 90 degrees again, and this time, gently pull your foot to your bottom. You can breathe out, hollow and zip, and then stretch for 20 to 30 seconds.

Hams Stretch
Exercise 11 in appendix.

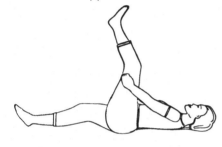

- Lie on your back.
- Straighten out one leg.
- Gently reach toward your straight leg (avoid this if you have back problems).
- If you do have a back issue, lie on your back with your knees bent. Hook your hand under your knee and straighten your leg a little then swap. Control with hollowing to protect your back.

You can do a straight leg stretch without back problems, just hold pain-free at end range for 20 to 30 seconds.

Calf Stretch
Exercise 41 in appendix.

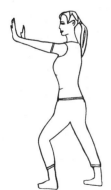

For the calf stretch, place one leg behind the other, with the knee bent. Then, straighten the knee slowly to feel comfortable, and stretch in the calf gently.

Abductor

Exercise 12 in appendix. Remove weight for the stretch.

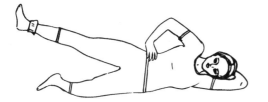

For this, do the above, then:

- Have your upper knee about six inches above the floor.
- Straighten out your knee, flex your ankle, and turn your toes down slightly.
- Lift your upper leg another six inches as you breathe out and pull in your belly button to protect your back.
- Breathe in as you lower your leg and repeat about a dozen times before putting your leg down and turning over.

Exercise 34 in appendix.

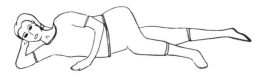

- Now, bend your upper leg and stretch out your lower leg.
- Push the top leg in front of the body and rest it.
- Hollow and contract your pelvic floor, breathing in as you lower to protect your back.
- Lift your lower leg up and move gently up and down to six inches above the floor, for 12 to 20 times maximum.
- You can stretch it out in this position.

Setting Your Fitness Goals

Patients often ask me, once their general fitness is much better, "How do I take the next step to train towards a specific sport?" Firstly, any current injuries should be assessed by a chartered physiotherapist. Then, you need to decide on your goals. What are your goals? Stronger heart and lungs? A fit looking body? To win at sport? To live longer? Furthermore, you need to decide: which sports you want to concentrate on, how vigorously you want to compete, and for how long you want to be able to compete.

Everyone should exercise, but you need to set your personal goals of fitness and your own unique set of aims, as this will determine the most appropriate exercise productive time you can spare for training. A fitness assessment with a personal trainer can establish your personal fitness goals and an injury prevention programme can be formulated to attain your goals of:

- Enhanced cardiovascular ability.
- Improved stamina and endurance.
- Better agility, flexibility, and balance.
- Stronger muscles and core strength.
- Slimmer body.
- Stronger bones.
- Clearer thinking and happier moods.

Ten Tips to Achieve Your Goals

1) Measure your heart rate just after vigorous exercise for 5 seconds, then after another minute for another 5 seconds. Multiply both by 12, then subtract one from the other. This gives you your speed of recovery, which is an indicator of your cardio fitness. As you get fitter, both your oxygen capacity and the ability of your enzymes to remove lactic acid will increase.

2) Mix up slow and fast pace in all activities. Athletes carry out long slow and short fast interval training for a good reason; the slow pace builds stamina and teaches the body how to cope with and eliminate lactic acid, as well as enabling muscles to store more glycogen for prolonged exercise.

3) Fast pace, on the other hand, comprises of short bursts of intense activity which boosts sugar metabolism and teaches the brain to co-ordinate the muscles at a faster pace, helping agility.

4) To avoid muscle injury due to tiredness, rest adequately as muscles need 48 hours to recover, plus good hydration and nutrition.

5) To achieve stronger muscles, lift a weight you can just manage between 8 and 12 lifts in about 50 seconds. Then, rest briefly between sets, as lactic acid build up will cause injury. Repeat. Rest a day in between. Add 2.5 kg to 5 kg maximum at each increase.

6) Exercised bones get stronger, so use resistance or weight bearing exercises.

7) For a thinner body, sustained exertion will burn up calories and speed up the metabolic rate.

8) For a flexible body, complete slow, sustained stretches of 30 seconds when you are warm and pain-free. Stretch before your workout to reduce the chances of injury. Stretching after exercise reduces muscle soreness and promotes relaxation.

9) Clearer thinking is essential. Work out your pattern of mental alertness, the daily peaks and troughs. Plan a regular exercise programme and see how it eliminates the 'valleys'. Exercise induced endorphins plus serotonin will reduce depression and pain.

10) For running, cycling and walking, get checked out biomechanically. This means the alignment of foot joints on the knees, hips, and back. Correct alignment will reduce wear and tear.

Recent research has shown that around 30% of the UK – that's a staggering 22 million people – suffer a sporting injury every year. So, if you decide to commit to a sporting profession, the chances are high that you will suffer multiple injuries over your career. In fact, you will pick up one to two injuries per year and take up to five days off work every year. There are even worse statistics as well: of all the people injured, 25% will not be able to carry on playing sport as a direct result of their sporting injury. If you love your sport, want to keep playing, and can't afford the risk of time off work, then you need to be proactive, making sure you know how to be as well prepared as you can be and knowing where to get the best treatment, so that if you are injured, you can get back to full fitness as quickly as possible.

Exercise is not, however, a substitute for physical treatment, as you'll find out in my next book, *The Human Garage*. Exercise is an integral part of keeping our muscles and bones healthy, and it is a necessary addition, but it isn't a substitute – and it never will be – for hands on physical therapy, acupuncture, diet, and revolutionary electrotherapy treatments to heal cellular destruction caused by injury and arthritis. Although, of course, current political behaviour is suggesting hands off exercise is the answer to pain, and is happy to add a cocktail of toxic pain killers into the already fragile tissue. If you are suffering nerve pain, for example, exercise can make you worse before treatment. Do not be a lemming; seek advice if you are in pain before pushing through that pain into further tissue destruction.

What does research say about time spent on exercise? Here's some more heavy science for you academic buffs! Half an hour a day may be quoted for being good for general health in the national guidelines, but it's not enough to ensure optimal health, and with our current food consumption, half an hour a day will not stop us from being fat. In fact, there is a fatty epidemic. Now, Australia's National Health and Medical Research Council (NHMRC) has suggested that daily activity needs to be doubled to an hour just to fight the nation's growing weight problem – unless we make big changes to what we eat. 'In the current environment of abundant availability, promotion and consumption of energy-dense food, it is now internationally recommended that 45 to 60 minutes of moderate-intensity daily physical activity is the minimum required... without reduction in current energy intake,' the NHMRC writes in its newly released report, Eat For Health (in 2014). 'At least 60 to 90 minutes of moderate-intensity activity (a day) or lesser amounts of vigorous activity may be required to prevent weight regain in formerly obese people,' it says. Who prescribes exercise? It has to come from you.

Message to the Doctors

Now here's a message to the doctors out there – you need to get fit to sell fitness. Recent research found that physically fit doctors were more likely to push for physical activity in patients than inactive doctors. Because people often take their doctor's advice seriously, 'these findings suggest that improving health care providers' physical activity levels may be an easy way to help reduce physical inactivity among the general population,' Isabel Garcia de Quevedo, of the U.S. Centers for Disease Control and Prevention, said in an American Heart Association news release (Furhman, 2000).

The study was presented recently at a meeting of the American Heart Association in New Orleans, and findings presented at medical meetings are typically considered preliminary until published in a peer-reviewed journal. The research team analysed the findings of 28 previous studies on health care providers' physical activity and the exercise counselling they gave to their patients. The review revealed that physically active health care providers were much more likely to advise their patients to get daily exercise.

Some of the studies found that fit, active doctors were two to five times more likely than inactive doctors to recommend exercise to their patients, while other studies found that programmes to improve doctors' physical activity levels improved the doctors' confidence and ability to provide exercise advice to patients. The researchers also discovered that medical school students who took part in a programme to improve their lifestyle habits were 56% more likely than other medical students to provide patients with regular physical activity counselling.

'When [exercise] advice is coupled with a referral to community resources, it can be quite effective and this approach should be part of the public health solution to America's inactivity problem,' study leader and co-author Dr. Felipe Lobelo, an epidemiologist with CDC's National Center for Chronic Disease Prevention and Health Promotion, said in the news release. 'The American Heart Association and the CDC recommend at least 150 minutes of moderate exercise or 75 minutes of vigorous exercise per week.' The U.S. National Heart, Lung and Blood institute offers a guide to physical activity.

Exercising from a young age improves cognitive function in later life, according to a new study from King's College London. Researchers analysed data on more than 9,000 British men and women who were followed by the 1958 National Child Development Study. They found that people performed better in mental tests at age 50 if they had engaged in regular intense exercise – such as running, swimming, or working out in the gym – since childhood.

Dr Alex Dregan, who led the study, believes that the findings support the need for a lifelong approach to improving cognitive ability, especially given growing public health concerns over the UK's ageing population. He said: 'As exercise represents a key component of lifestyle interventions to prevent cognitive decline, cardiovascular disease, diabetes, and cancer, public health interventions to promote lifelong exercise have the potential to reduce the personal and social burden associated with these conditions in late adult years.' The government recommends that adults aged between 19 and 64 should exercise for at least 150 minutes per week.

However, the study indicated that even exercising less frequently than this may help to improve cognitive function. For example, people who exercised just once a week as a child and adult performed better on tests of memory, learning, attention, and reasoning at age 50 compared to those who did not. The study's findings also suggest that intense physical activity may offer greater benefits for brain function in later life than less intense but regular exercise; the researchers found a gradual increase in memory scores with higher intensity exercise.

'It's widely acknowledged that a healthy body equals a healthy mind. However, not everyone is willing or able to take part in the recommended 150 minutes of physical activity per week,' Dr Dregan said. 'For these people, any level of physical activity may benefit their cognitive wellbeing in the long-term and this is something that needs to be explored further. Setting lower exercise targets at the beginning and gradually increasing their frequency and intensity could be a more effective method for improving levels of exercise within the wider population' (Dregan and Gulliford, 2013).

The Power of Posture

This is an important activity to carry through into a lifestyle change, as good posture helps maintain a healthy mind and body, and when you correct your posture on a daily basis, your body is in much better alignment. Changing our posture also changes our mindset; have you ever met an upright individual striding out and shouting, "I am so depressed"? Good posture is taught at my clinic in order to avoid painful muscle contractures and to protect nerves, and it is also the essence of preventative care for your joints. Do you stand with even weight through your legs? Get out two pairs of scales and see: look at the reading through each leg. Are you evenly balanced? As you bring awareness and gain better posture, take a picture of yourself and draw around the outline. Standing, walking, and sitting correctly can help to alleviate common problems such as back and neck pain, headaches, and low moods.

Mirror Mirror on the Wall, Who Is...

Using a mirror, stand tall, with your weight evenly balanced through both feet, and gently rock forward and back. Imagine a rope through the top of your head, lining up with your ears, your shoulders and then your hips (proper alignment places your ears in line with your shoulders and hips). These points ideally should be in a straight line and can be sketched on the wall – the spine should be a gently curving S shape. Take a picture on your phone, side on. How upright are you?

Are You Sitting Comfortably? Then I Will Begin
Exercise 17 in appendix.

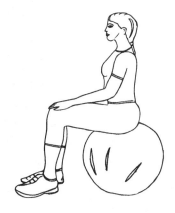

If, like myself when I am writing, you need to spend hours at a desk, use a chair that is ergonomically designed for your height and weight. If this is not an option, try using a small pillow for lumbar support. I sit on a fitball when I can, and get up and stretch regularly. Align yourself with the back of the chair, and don't lean back or forward too much. Adjust your chair and your position so your arms are flexed, not straight out, and aim roughly for a 75 to 90 degree angle at the elbows. Work your core muscles regularly by contracting your tummy and pelvic floor. Practise slow tummy breathing, three breaths every half an hour. As with standing posture, keep your shoulders squared up, head upright, on top of your neck. Both feet should be flat on the floor, with your heels, back, and neck in line.

When Driving

Keep your eyes on the road (haha), your back against the seat, and your neck against the head rest. Adjust your seat to maintain a proper distance from the pedals and the steering wheel – if you are bunched up with your chin on top of the steering wheel, you are too close. If leaning forward, you are too far away from the wheel. Adjust the head rest so it is reasonably close to the back of your head.

Sleeping

If you prefer to lie on your side, try slipping a cushion between your legs to help keep your spine aligned. Use a curved single pillow at the correct height to fill the space between your ear and your shoulder. Get advice on the type of mattress and pillow you should be using.

Walk Tall

We are not designed to walk on hard ground; if the way our foot moves over the ground is less than perfect, premature ageing occurs in our weight-bearing joints and spine. To assess this scientifically needs biomechanical analysis, with gait scanning technology. I personally find it a great tool in the clinic to predict and alleviate problems in the feet, ankles, knees, hips, and spine. Then, wear and tear through all the lower limb joints and spine can be lessened with muscle strengthening, correct shoe wear, and possibly precision-made orthotics. Learn to walk in an anti-ageing way, correctly and softly on hard ground.

Learning To Walk Again – Good Posture in Walking

Using resistive exercises gives a more elastic gait and helps weight control, and something as simple as ankle weights can help. For example, putting on an extra 20 lbs of muscle will consume about an extra 120 calories, about the same as a 10 minute workout. If you want to use your upper limbs more, try Nordic walking, which I will return to later.

Exercise 40 in appendix.

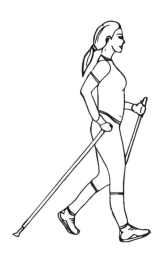

How about I teach you how to walk like a celebrity? Let's start. Feel the ground through your heels – 80% of your weight should go through your heels. Now, soften your knees to take the pull off your hamstrings (the muscles at the backs of your thighs), and gently tense your stomach muscles and pelvic floor, as this aligns the pelvis and adjusts the breastbone. Then, rest your shoulders into position with a roll back action, and remember – the ears should be above your shoulders, and by moving your head back and forth, you can sit your head on top. This should set you up for a healthy spine through walking. Now, please avoid these three key mistakes. If you walk flat-footed, you can get bunions and a bad back from it. Add in big steps and you can get chronic knee cap problems – which are common in runners – and this can lead to a bad back as your natural lordotic curve increases and destabilises the lumbar spine. If you lock your knees out on stepping, your knees suffer and the back overarches again.

Let's do my favourite walking exercise together right now. Slow down your steps – those old enough to remember the bionic man know what I mean. If you slow down your steps, taking seconds to place one foot in front of the other, it enables you to correct bad habits. Heel strike slowly without immediate weight, and feel how it keeps the step shorter and how it will give you more stability. Gently be aware of how you drop your tailbone and rotate your hip, as the weight transfers through your foot to your toe, and the back foot easily lifts off as the weight is transferred. These baby steps are an example of the type of exercises that elite athletes return to time and again to keep elasticity/the spring in their step. Add in ankle weights – as you see me at work doing from time to time – and your youthful appearance is born.

Now, here's some research to back up my love of speed walking: in 2013, a study outlined how speed walking is said to be one of the most effective back pain treatments. 'Although physicians recommend that patients suffering from back pain engage in proper diet and regular exercise, there is still a need to specifically address certain activities that may result in significant pain relief. A recent medical report published in the journal Pain Research and Treatment showed that walking can decrease the intensity of back pain, and more importantly, walking at higher speed can result in more enhanced pain relief.' (This was by the Department of Physical Education and Sports Sciences, University of Mohaghegh Ardabili, Iran).

I believe that fitness and wellness go hand-in-hand; if our bodies are fit, then we are supporting a healthy mind, free to concentrate on the pleasures of life. Mankind has recognised this link for thousands of years, even going back to the time of Hippocrates; 'if we give every individual the right amount of nourishment and exercise, not too little and not too much, we would have found the safest way to health.' Ongoing extensive research has proven that Hippocrates' instincts were correct: we now know scientifically that exercise is effective in lessening the risk of arthritis, heart disease, cancer, osteoporosis, diabetes, depression, brain deterioration, and in reducing stress.

Recent studies have shown that if you engage in regular activity and spend less time in front of the TV, you will benefit from a more positive outlook, better weight control, a good boost to your immune system, and a healthier, longer life. Research from America, at the veterans' hospital in Boston, made the same link: if you increase your activity, you can add seven years to your life. It is also especially important to keep fit as you get older, when there is a tendency to slow down. We can all feel the buzz exercise gives us, and what we probably don't realise is that sufficient exercise reduces stress. Going one stage further, very recent research has implicated stress as a culprit to DNA damage, and even worse, the consequences of parental stress can be passed down to our children.

So how can you achieve a fit body with a busy lifestyle? You need to listen to your body, understanding how much movement your body craves and how long to rest for when fatigue hits. Also, if you increase your level of activity, make sure your cells receive more fluids and more minerals.

Five Top Tips to Everyday Fitness

1) If you drive a car for more than an hour or two, break the journey up and take a walk._Park away from your destination and take the time to walk briskly, swinging your arms. This will ease the pressure on your spinal discs, loosen stiffened joints and improve blood flow.

2) Make sure your shoes fit well. If you have been prescribed orthotics, wear them. When we do our biomechanics assessments, it is surprising how often they are needed. When you walk, allow your body to glide with even, flowing, quiet footsteps. Then, gradually build up the pace to power walk for at least ten minutes a day.

3) If you work at a desk, swap your chair for a fitball. The small movements keep your mind focused and your spine healthy.

4) Take your fitball away from the desk, and do a workout on it for ten minutes, twice a day. By adding in a pilates move of gently pulling in your tummy button to your spine, you will sit for longer and more comfortably.

5) Follow a weekly plan of activity, like mine listed below. If you wish to achieve a steady progression of fitness, or get fit for a holiday or sports activity, ask the guidance of a personal fitness instructor. We have Dean at the clinic to help keep us trim.

Example of a 7 Day Fitness Programme

This is suitable for those working full-time. I work full-time myself, plus I teach, write, run a business, and see patients over seven days, which means that exercise has to be a discipline. This evolves all the time, and the discipline of putting the time aside is the secret here.

Saturday/Sunday – Aerobic Workout

I jog or cycle outside for at least half an hour to an hour, if not exercising at the gym or swimming. My favourite place to do this is on a sandy beach on a hot, sunny day.

Monday to Friday – Aerobic Workout

Five days a week, I will go for a jog for over 45 minutes with interval training and power walking, and I swim three to five times a week for 30 minutes, again with interval training. Three times a week I do resistive exercises at the gym or at home, using weights for 20 to 30 minutes (see section on weights workout), and I warm up with the treadmill, cycle, stepper, or rower to raise my heart rate over 10 minutes. Five evenings a week, I do 15 minutes of stretching and meditation with vital exercises such as yoga or chi kung, as well as a core workout, or I do a Western workout of fitball, stretches, and core work for 15 to 30 minutes at home or my clinic, whilst listening to inspiring CDs or business tapes.

Fitball

Exercise 17 in appendix.

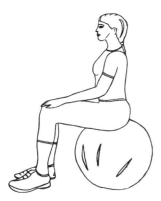

I enjoy my fitballs; I sit on the larger ones at my desks and use the smaller ones for exercising – the size you need to choose depends on your height and leg length. It's a great workout tool, if you use it correctly to reap the benefits, and it's great to add versatility to your exercises.

In the 1980s in Switzerland and the USA, the fitball was used for rehabilitation of injuries and for chronic debilitating conditions. I go to refresh my exercises at my friend and practice manager's fitball class at my favourite haunt, Hoar Cross Hall. I pant and giggle through my abdominal and spine workout, and my leg and arm strengthening exercises – it's great to work on my proprioception to improve my stance and posture and to protect my joints. If I sit at my desk on a fitball, it improves my posture and alleviates back pain by not stressing the small postural muscles so much and protecting the discs with better alignment.

Exercise 16 in appendix.

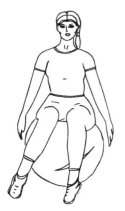

You can use your pilates breathing, sitting well onto the ball, and do the zip up pelvic floor exercise. Then, you can add in limb movements and stomach work as directed by your teacher. It's great to do a few exercises – say 15 – a day, progressing the ability as you go.

Fitball Bridge

Exercise 18 in appendix.

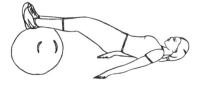

- Rest your ankles on the ball whilst lying on your back.
- Do a tummy pilates breath and lift your bottom off the floor.

I like using it for all sorts, especially the bridge after sitting for a while. Don't attempt this exercise if your back is sore, though.

Vital Energy Exercises – The Eastern Way to Keep Healthy

'One should rely half on the doctor and half on the shaman'
(The Okinawa Way)

I want to write about exercise that has an impact on our health in terms of improving vitality, and in Eastern terms, when we talk about vital energy we're talking about the chi factor. I came across such a strong cultural tie to ancient ways of exercising out in China town in Vancouver, in China itself, and in Korea. My own personal roots in Eastern medicine started with my lecturing years in the early 2000s, talking about dry needling, as taught by my Malaysian master.

Energy is called chi in china, ki in Japan, and prana in India, and this effect of generating chi can be experienced by doing breathing exercises and meditation with yoga, tai chi, and qigong. In Chinese medicine, chi is either material or immaterial: the former can be gained through raw food, ionised water, and air, and for the latter – the immaterial – it is said that we are born with a reserve that responds to conscious exercise.

Tai Chi

Exercise 15 in appendix.

Another vitality exercise is tai chi, and its precise, flowing movements stem from martial arts. You develop better posture and strength through this 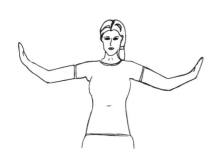 discipline and it also brings inner calmness, another bonus. I enjoyed these classes and I was often put at the front so I couldn't cheat and follow someone in front of me – it takes some concentration! It also needs the discipline of practise, and at the time I was also studying dance, so I decided to return later to this discipline. Students learn a basic sequence of movements: a short form for beginners and a more involved form for those who are more experienced.

Tai chi is a moving form of meditation, with the student being aware of chi moving in the body, and it is also a soft martial art, developing a flexible, controlled, balanced mind and body. My Malaysian professor would prescribe me tai chi exercises, saying that out in rural China or Malaysia, farmers were often illiterate – however, they could move like a tiger or bird, mimicking the movements of the animals, which is what tai chi is modelled after.

Tai chi is a more modern derivative of chi kung, an old Chinese art, with its softness building up inner power within a flexible body. The Japanese government adapted some of its movements for a nationwide exercise programme aimed at promoting fitness. This is part of the ongoing Radio Taiso, and every day in the morning, millions of Japanese exercise to this. Medical exams show that the benefits are akin to Western aerobic exercise, without stress and strains through joints. Tai chi helps depression, muscle tension, rehab post heart surgery, high and low BP, chronic illness, rheumatoid and osteoarthritis, stress-related insomnia, and spines and bones generally.

One of my patients runs a class close to the clinic. On my first consultation, she was on crutches, but last week she ran in for her massage with a colleague, and showed everyone – at age 71 – how easy it was to lift her leg over the reception counter. Her joints are great and for a rheumatoid arthritic patient, that is amazing. She told me of one study of 256 inactive people aged 70 to 92, who took up tai chi. This group fell half as much as a group who stretched only. Considering that after age 75, falls are the main cause of unexpected death, that's impressive.

A lot of research has been carried out on Eastern exercise by the FICSIT (Frailty and Injuries Coop Studies of Intervention Techniques) and the NIA (the U.S. National Institute on Aging). Several studies showed a reduction in falls, improved grip strength, lowered BP, increased confidence, and mobility (Lai, Lan, and Wong et al., 1995, Wolfson, Whipple, and Derby et al., 1996, Kessenich, 1998, and Lane and Nydick, 1999).

There are several more studies to back this up. For instance, 20 males and females aged 58 to 70 practised three to six sessions of tai chi a week over an average of 24 minutes. Their fitness increased by 19%, their spine flexibility by 10%, and their leg length by 18% (Lan, Lai, and Chen et al., 1998). It also helps my arthritic patients. Generally, it is an evidence-based, cost effective, therapeutic exercise (Yocum, Castro, and Corne, 2000).

Get a teacher to demonstrate the form for you. You need a good 10 square feet of floor space, and due to the slow, flowing movements used, make sure you're dressed in unrestrictive clothing. Have relaxed, slightly flexed knees and elbows, and then rotate the head to be in line with the body. The movements are said to cleanse the meridian lines and renew healing processes, and they also still the chattering monkey mind. I used to like standing at the back of the class as I tended to forget the odd bit.

Exercises 22 and 23 in appendix.

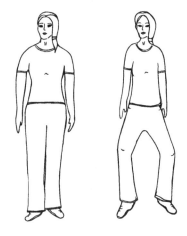

Here's perhaps one of my favourite movements and an easy one to start with. Stand and centre yourself, with your knees straight and your arms by your side. Imagine being suspended by a thread from the heavens, through your body and to the earth. Empty your thoughts and repeat an inspiring mantra. Stand with your feet together and your weight evenly distributed through your feet, then relax and soften your knees.

Inhale through your nose, into your tummy – this focuses chi – and then raise your arms slowly, with your fingers hanging loose, like they are floating in water. Hold your breath for a couple of seconds, then exhale and lower your arms, with your wrists held up slightly and flexed gently as you float them down. This is just a taster of the start of an inspiring routine – go and find a class and enjoy.

Chi Kung or Qigong

Chi means energy, while kung means art, and chi kung together refers to the art of developing life energy for health, internal power, mind, and spirit. I was interested in vitality exercises that worked with meridians, having studied Chinese acupuncture and shiatsu (Japanese physio), as well as my years of reiki training, which helped me to feel subtle energy changes as well as physical ones.

In the 1960s, Liu Gui Zhen used chi kung to treat chronic degenerative disease, and like with my reiki master training, you can transmit healing thoughts over long distances. At an advanced level, it is taught in a spiritual as well as physical way, and it is divided into different aspects: medical, martial, Confucianist, Taoist, and Buddhist. Chinese records of chi kung have been found as far back as 2,700 BCE. In the 3rd century, Buddhist meditation influenced chi kung, and those aspects are classified as being from the Buddhist school. In the 7th century, Tang Dynasty martial arts masters also made use of chi kung, hence the martial school of chi kung. The 13th century saw tai chi chaun, while the 17th century saw pakua and hsing yi, all different styles. Neo Confucianism gained popularity since the 10th century, while the Taoist school of chi kung is noted for its visualisation and breathing techniques.

When I was out in China, exploring Chinese history, it was incredible to see so much historical evidence that you could still touch, which went back centuries. I would turn a corner and there would be more treasures, more palaces, the terracotta army, and so on. Chi kung is so much more than breathing and gentle exercises; it expands your creative imagination and feeds the soul, and it is much more still and centred than other vital energy exercises. In fact, the Taoist secrets of conserving sexual energy came from these disciplines, and these modern day masters breathe very efficiently and their circulation is much better. Beyond the physical, the peace they emanate is beautiful, and this comes from the discipline of the art, of staying young and tolerant of others. It is said to be helpful in blood pressure problems, as well as with asthma, insomnia, arthritis, migraine, diabetes, and kidney problems, to name a few.

Chi kung has four parts: dynamic, self-manifested chi, quiescent chi kung, and meditation. The objectives with dynamic can be to help with disease for preventative health or more flexibility. Self-manifested chi features a group of exercises that allow you to enjoy flowing meditation through movement, and using breath is very much a chi kung art. The most popular is abdominal, creating a pearl of energy at this point to spread to any part of the body, and the vital centre of the body is the kath – point three finger breadths below the belly button and 2.5 cm inwards to find it. Diakath breathing concentrates on filling the lungs up from the bottom to the top and emptying from the top to the bottom, using nine breaths per session. Cosmic energy is said to be trapped at the qihai, or the kath point.

Many other breathing techniques have names: reverse breath is when an explosive action or punch is needed, while cosmic breath in the chest is to tap cosmic energy to store in the abdomen. Others include foetal breath for being passive, tortoise breath for longevity, and heel to breathe into the heels. Small universe breathing is when kung fu fighters keep chi flowing through ren and du meridians, while big universe breathing focuses on chi through the meridian channels – this is employed by Taoist masters to train immortality. 'No breathing' by masters is when vital meets cosmic to attain enlightenment – I experienced the struggle to breathe when you feel so still in that spiritual place. The Chinese spoke of breathing in energy and we in the West translated it later to air.

Meditation in chi kung can be very advanced and deeply spiritual, and patience is most definitely needed. I currently enjoy the shaolin wahnam chi kung patterns, and the first ten of these dynamic movements are a good starting point. Buy a book, find a master, and enjoy. This a blend of Zen Buddhism and kung fu. In terms of the actual exercises, I will describe just one in detail.

Lifting the Sky
Exercises 19, 20, and 15 in appendix.

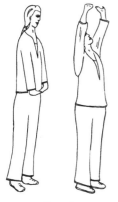 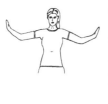

This is said to be one of the best exercises in chi kung, and you should do this while smiling through the heart. If it is the only exercise you are doing, repeat many times – say 21.

- Stand with your feet together and your arms down.
- Make sure that your arms are straight and that your fingertips are pointing inwards, towards each other.
- Gently move your arms up and visualise cosmic energy flowing into you.
- Reach up and push up at the sky, with your wrists at 90 degrees.
- Then bring your arms down again, like birds' wings.
- Whilst bringing your arms down, imagine any negative thoughts and illness going away.

Other exercises in this group include the plucking star, pushing mountains, carrying the moon, circulating head, merry go round, big windmill, hula hoop, and deep knee bending. You need to ideally find a tutor to demo these, or at least see a video, before attempting them yourself.

Yoga

My third vitality exercise I want to talk about is yoga, and yoga in itself is a huge subject. Unlike chi kung, yoga puts more emphasis on stretching and posture and less on keeping still and feeling energy. Chi kung is more famous for stress control and sexual Taoist energy with anti-ageing powers, but there is, however, a lot of cross over. Archaeological evidence of ancient statues places this art at 5,000 years old, and yoga has many forms, some more physical and some more spiritual, in order to gain enlightenment.

Yoga is from the language of ancient India, and it means 'union'. The feeling of wellbeing is gained by connecting breathing with stretches, believed to also have an impact on the internal organs. This is a great way to relax and improve your posture all at the same time, although greater balance and better, stronger core muscles are needed to achieve many of the postures. Relieving mental stress on a regular basis improves immunity, and breathing – as mentioned in my mindset chapter – links with emotional and cardiovascular health, BP, and lung function. Good posture relieves back pain, whereas the calming poses and breathing help to alleviate stress, and there is a lot of scientific evidence to back up these claims (such as in Shealy's alternative medicine encyclopaedia).

Morning, they say, is often seen as the best time to exercise, although I often do some at night to unwind, due to the clinical hours that I work. You need to always dress in soft clothing, with bare feet and not too much food in your stomach. A towel, mat, cushion, and bathing rope are useful tools to help ease tight joints and to allow for a gentler stretch, especially as a beginner or if you have damaged joints or irritated nerves. Slow, gentle, flowing, pain-free movements are the safest. As I've said, there are many versions of yoga – some more focused on the physical, with others more focused on the spiritual, which include more meditation.

So when did yoga start getting so popular in the West? Swami Vivekananda came to the USA in the 1890s, and this was when yoga was born in the West, as a gentle exercise that uses breathing to bridge the mind with the body and enables flexibility to be maintained in later years. A review of twenty years' worth of scientific studies, conducted by researchers at Duke University Medical Center, found that yoga is effective in the treatment of chronic pain, including osteoarthritis, carpal tunnel syndrome, and fibromyalgia. In the studies reviewed, patients saw significant reductions in joint pain, muscle stiffness, and overall physical discomfort while greatly improving their flexibility, range of motion, and muscle strength.

Why Yoga?
Exercise 37 in appendix.

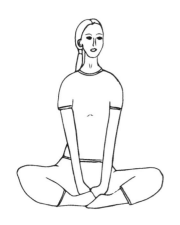

With yoga, the goal is to exercise in an intuitive, centred, calm and connected spiritual way. Feeling movement in an easy way is a nice sensation, especially when you want to get in a mindset to relax, focus on creative writing, or wind down in the evenings. You can still get a sweat up and tone muscles without going at it like a bull at a gate, and it is quite a skill to be able to relax the facial muscles and mind whilst working the body. It's a great tool to practise feeling good about your body and sensitising the movements to build awareness of you, about how you feel concerning all aspects of your life, and how your posture reflects this. This awareness builds with time and is empowering and liberating about who you are and who you want to be.

Performed correctly, yoga has great physical benefits, as yoga's fluid movements allow swollen or otherwise painful joints to glide smoothly over one another, increasing mobility and strength without excess wear and tear.

It was a pleasure to watch my very experienced co-presenter at Z factor, Goedele Leyssen, demonstrate yoga beautifully, especially her special take on Kundalini yoga. This ancient practice comes in so many forms.

Of course, before performing any of the below pain relieving poses, be sure to talk with your therapist first about any injuries you may have and use props such as blocks for support as needed. Here is just a handful of some of my beginner poses that I do at home. Thanks to Goedele for inspiring me and to the classes at HXH (Hoar Cross Hall) for reminding me how inflexible I can be compared to the gurus in this art.

Yoga Pose: The Cobra
Exercise 27 in appendix.

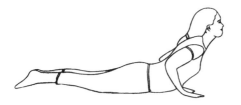

This is nice to stretch out backs, but take care if you have arthritis in the facet joints. I do this when I am writing a lot. Lie face down, with your forehead resting on the floor. Place your hands on the middle of your ribcage, one at either side. Then draw your legs together, resting the tops of your feet onto the floor. You can then let your heels turn out and press through your hands as you draw your elbows close to your ribcage. Using the strength of your back (*not arms*), lift your head and chest, sliding your shoulder blades down your back. You can rest on your forearms, or if comfortable, take it into an extended elbow stretch, keeping your pelvis on the floor. Take five slow, deep breaths, hollowing your stomach before gently releasing to the floor.

Yoga Pose: The Cat
Exercise 04 in appendix.

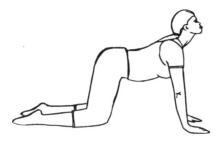

I like to go from this position to the cat – it sounds politer than the doggie positon! The cat has you place your hands under your shoulder with your knees under your hips, and then

176

breathe in as you lift your head, ears, and tail, and push your middle back to earth – mewing is optional.

Yoga Pose: Supported Warrior

Exercise 41 in appendix.

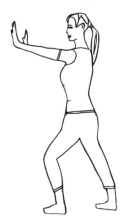

This exercise allows you to stretch out your calves and work your knees – I like this as I am flat-footed and my calves get tight. Stand tall and place your hands against a wall at shoulder height. Step with your right foot forward so your toes touch the wall, and bend your knee at 90 degrees, bending your elbows behind as though you're trying to push the wall away. Step with your left foot about a couple of feet behind you, slightly bending your left knee. Hold for 10 breaths and tummy hollows, then, slowly straighten your left leg while bending your right knee, taking care of too much stretch in your achilles. Hold for 10 breaths again before stepping with your left foot forward to meet the right, then switch leg positions. You can go into warrior lift or reverse warrior by raising your arms.

Yoga Pose: Butterfly

Exercise 2 in appendix.

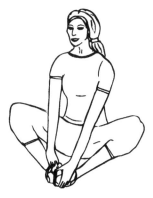

Sitting down, bring the soles of your feet together, with your knees wide so your legs form a shape resembling butterfly wings. Keep your entire back straight and your shoulders relaxed as you breathe and gently drop weight off the legs, slowly allowing your knees to lower toward the floor. For gentler relief, place blocks or pillows beneath your outer knees for support as well as under your bottom. This is an alternative to the adductor stretch position.

Exercise 36 in appendix.

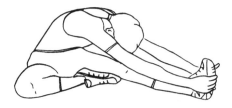

Then, straighten your legs out in front of you, placing the sole of your left foot against the inside of your right leg. Reach gently towards your foot, then swap legs.

Head to Knee Forward Bend
Exercise 24 in appendix.

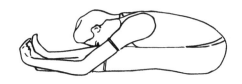

Straighten your legs out and loop the Theraband belt around your feet, stretching your hams towards your feet. Hold with a breath and do hollow tummy work.

Yoga Sitting Pose
Exercise 37 in appendix.

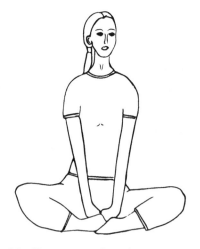

Going back into a seated posture with crossed knees, I like to go through my thoracic rotation stretches, with my arms behind my back, stretching and going up over the head. I need my Thoracic and shoulder stretching routine when I have been writing for too long. Place a folded towel under your bum and bring the soles of your feet together, with your legs in the butterfly position. Breathe and hollow tum, then lower your shoulder blades and breathe in and out. With your hands on your ankles, let your knees move up and down, before crossing your ankles, hollowing your tum, and placing your hands on your shoulders. Then, with your elbows together, draw a circle with them, before extending your elbows and clasping your hands from your chin to chest – stretch them out and then up. Release and stretch behind you, then stretch your right arm to the ceiling and bend your elbow as if to scratch your back, holding a piece of Theraband or towel between your hands in this position and gently moving your hands together and swapping sides. Then, put your left hand to your right knee and your right hand behind your back, before doing a slow twist and untwist.

Standing Mountain Pose

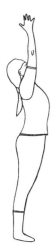

When I am feeling overwhelmed, I kick off my shoes, close my eyes, and stand, observing like the watcher within any swaying movements. For the standing mountain pose, stand and take your arms up while breathing in.

Exercise 26 in appendix.

Standing Tree Pose

This is useful when working on standing posture and weight transfer. With your legs together, gently hollow your tum. Place your weight on the toes of your feet and then the heels, before transferring the weight to your right leg. Place the sole of your left foot lightly on the right. Take your arms up into a prayer position, breathe and relax, then lower your arms and place the weight back through both feet. If you have good balance, you can place the sole of your foot on your inner thigh – not a good idea, however, if you are near expensive pottery. I then open my eyes, straighten my arms above my head, and look upwards, taking slow deep breaths, before opening my arms into a V shape. This is also called the Standing Arm Reach. If you can link hands and stretch left and right above your head like a tree swaying, it's called Standing Sidebend.

Standing Forward Bend
Exercise 42 in appendix.

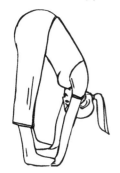

Then I reach down and hang there, breathing out and stretching out my lower back and hams – very soothing after a run. I stand again then repeat, bending my knees slightly, before bending over and gently hanging there, allowing a soothing lengthening in the spine. Then I hollow and uncurl gently, until standing again.

Yoga Standing Pose: Wall Plank, Strengthening Arms
Exercise 41 in appendix.

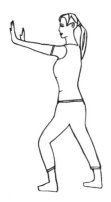

Stand facing the wall with your feet hip-width apart, not against a door like my patients try to do in my office – not good news for your nose. Place your palms against the wall, with your arms extended, and slowly lean forward, letting your body rest on your hands. Keep your arms in and your body in a straight line as you slowly bend your elbows, inching closer to the wall. When you feel discomfort, hollow your stomach, breathe out, and slowly push back to a standing position.

Yoga Standing Mudra Pose:
Arm Lift Behind You with Strap
Exercise 22 in appendix.

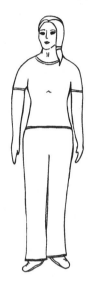

You cannot answer the phone in this position. Stand tall, with your feet apart, holding your Theraband or strap in one hand. Sweep both arms behind your back – with one above your head and one below – and then pull your shoulders in to grasp the strap with both hands in a comfortable position. Walk your hands carefully toward each other, opening your chest and stretching your pectorals as your shoulder blades move toward one another. Breathe and gently hollow your stomach as you adjust your shoulders, easing or increasing tension.

There are many different yoga forms. Briefly, here are the names:

- **Hatha yoga:** emphasises breathing control and holding positions.
- **Raja yoga**: meditation and mental being key here.
- **Ashtanga yoga:** links hatha strenuous positions with flowing movements and breathing control whilst moving, with some lock positions.
- **Tantric yoga:** to do with Kundalini and sexual awakening, but also brings in hatha element. Kundalini yoga is described as the coiled serpent, an energy yoga working with chakras.

Patients often say to me, "I can't get into meditation, I don't enjoy being still – it's irritating." Well, here's the answer: meditate whilst moving. It's basically the feeling of reflecting on thoughts as they pass softly through your mind, as you still from the chattering monkey, and it's a sensation of a space opening up inside you, a peaceful connection, a stillness, a place where anything is possible.

Once you have mastered slowing your mind with movement, still meditation is a smaller step. I love my CD that John Parker gave me at Z factor; John teaches meditation in such a soft, spiritual way, and his musical gifts make his voice so rhythmical and soothing. John went on to explain to me transcendental meditation and siddha, which work more deeply on the subconscious mind, switching off fight or flight responses.

Yoga Breath

Exercise 37 in appendix.

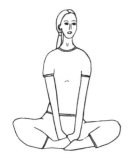

My God, there are so many! At Z factor, a Dutch girl, Goedelle showed us several and I made a few brief notes:

- **Basic yoga breath:** nose out, mouth in.
- **Box breath:** breathe in for 4 seconds, hold for 4 seconds, and out for 4 seconds.
- **Alternative nostril breath:** hand closes over other nostril.
- **Breath of fire:** forcing fast breath in and out through the nose.
- **Bellows breath:** big inhale, fast exhale.

You can also say mantras, like "it's time for a cuppa," – just kidding!

Pilates

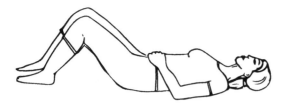

Exercise 3 in appendix.

Pilates is the fourth form of vitality exercise, which although very westernised in its form, has Eastern roots, so it needs to at least be mentioned here as well. In the West, this exercise was devised by a German sportsman, who was trained in wrestling, boxing, and gymnastics. He was interned during the First World War and designed the pilates regime, which he then went on to include in his dance training. Pilates employs low impact, slow controlled movements with breathing, and this strengthens the core and improves balance reactions and flexibility.

I see it as a fusion of yoga, core stability, and tai chi, and I find it especially helpful for patients with back problems, who have little ability to move and balance. Getting rid of bad posture gives grace to the way you sit and walk, and this improves your kinaesthetic sense, which controls the coordination of muscle contractions. Focusing on small, controlled movements enhances the sensitivity of the nervous system to enable us to perform everyday activities with grace. Correct posture lessens pain and ageing on our spinal discs and joints, and adding a fitball or Theraband helps to boost the toning effect of the muscles. I have taught elements of pilates to patients over the years, and I attend classes to put myself through my paces. I never fail to realise its importance and how short-lived our memory of good muscle control is.

To sum up, exercise and fitness could be many books' worth and this chapter is a whistle-stop tour of different types of exercise and why it's so important to move. Now, listen up! It's thoroughly illogical to believe that optimal fitness can be gained by an hour a day – what about the other 15 hours? Fitness is a lifestyle, not a daily task. You need to walk more and brisker, and every task is a good excuse to move and stretch into it. Silly things they might seem, but they are free and lifesaving, like jumping up and down while watching TV advert breaks, standing on one leg on the phone, sitting on a fitball, singing and shouting out loud, walking faster, using steps, and getting outside whenever you can – if you do these things, now you are extending your life.

For example, if you unsteady outside or have weak legs and don't know how to start exercising, Nordic walking means you can use 90% of your muscles – especially if chatting, ladies – and burn 50% more fat. It's good for spinal problems because it uses the abdominal muscles and upper body muscles, and it can also take some strain off recovering hips or knees. Poles are inexpensive, so make sure you add them to your fitness kit of heart rate monitor, pedometer, fitball, dumbbells, and Theraband.

Exercise that helps balance is critical as we get older – more about falling in lifestyle chapter. Falling over at 75+ is the leading cause of death. You can do little lifesaving exercises a few minutes every day, such as standing on one leg or walking heel to toe in a straight line – it will make a difference. Exercise needs to be a lifestyle change, and something which is considered at all waking hours. Find a hobby you are passionate about – preferably outside – that needs you to move. I don't mean get passionate outside; you may get arrested!

Do 30 to 60 minutes a day of aerobic exercises, ones that aim to work your heart and lungs and as many muscles as possible, such as Nordic walking, cycling, running, rowing, or aerobic classes. Do resistive exercises in a session three times a week to improve bone density, muscle function, and hormone levels. A flexibility workout is great, ideally every day, incorporating your favourite form e.g. yoga, Western stretches, pilates, or swimming. Also do some balance and anti-fall activities for a few minutes every day, please. Timetable this in for a month and then return to the questionnaire in the appendix.

Here's a fun scientific true fact: for men, a wank a day keeps the doctor away! Yes, that's right – masturbating once a day is known to reduce prostate cancer. In a study of 29,342 men aged 46 to 81, there were a third fewer cases (Reader's Digest, 2009). Something to think about.

As Hippocrates said, 'if we could give every individual the right amount of nourishment and exercise, not too little and not too much, we would have found the safest way to health.' So move guys – with a smile on your face.

———◦○◦———

Unrealistic Expectations Are Achievable –
You Can Bounce/Fly at Sixty

Paul is an intense sixty year old, who retired very early on from being a fireman. He had been to see many professionals, but no one could give him the body and sporting performance of a twenty-one year old, which is what he was striving for. So, when he came to see me, he let me know that my chances of failure were very high.

Fitness, he told me, was everything to him. He just had a need to run like an express train for twenty-five miles a day, cycle with the Tour de France team, and ski like an Olympian. Of course, this was all in between looking after his grandkids. He also wanted to get rid of the twinge of pain he got from his spondylotic neck, his lumbar spine, and his arthritic knee.

His health questionnaire answers were: diet – green. Mindset – green. Fitness – green. Lifestyle, relationships and work balance – green. He was, after all, retired and rich. On the surface, he had no problems whatsoever, but on closer examination, Paul had back rot, which was causing many of his issues.

Step One was to improve his alignment by looking at adjusting his biomechanics with orthotics. This meant that his 'heel to toe' could be better.

Step Two was to examine his fitness training. It was found that he needed better stretching and that he needed to focus on core strengthening work. Both his diet and hydration tests were excellent, and he was slim.

Step Three involved NLP (Neuro-linguistic Programming) to adjust his amazingly unrealistic expectations and to moderate his unrealistic beliefs about his spine and his fitness.

Step Four is where I agreed to take him on for the challenge of IMS, for both his lumbar and his neck. This eliminated muscle contractures.

Step Five saw him undergoing MBST/MRT for osteoarthritis in the knee and facet joints, as well as re-growing the balding areas of the cartilage. The results for this were excellent. He had no pain; he went up the Tour de France course, he went running, and he had no problems whatsoever. He also agreed to getting a regular sports massage close to home, as he was now north of twenty-one by forty years.

So was this a happy ending? Well, no, not quite...

It seemed that Paul thought he could fly – off a piste, in fact, which resulted in him bouncing on his head. He rang me in indignation from his hospital bed, informing me of what he'd done and complaining that he had his 'niggle' back. Well, within three weeks, he was back skiing with his niggle resolved, proving that you can, in fact, bounce at sixty.

The point of this story is that even seemingly unrealistic expectations can be achievable. The lesson I learnt here is that if you strive for optimum health and have a structured training programme which respects your body, you can still strive for sporting excellence and expect to get it, no matter what your age.

When Actors Need To Be Fit Too

We don't often think about how actors are feeling when they're portraying someone on screen, but it can be incredibly difficult if, for example, they're in immense pain but are playing a character who is not – it's not something you can easily hide, and the camera picks up on every wince and every pained expression.

Therefore, it shouldn't come as a surprise that sometimes actors seek out help when working on a project that needs to be pain-free. It was following one of my health columns in a monthly magazine that an actor contacted me about a neck injury, and 'Darling' was asked to be on call on set whilst a TV series was being filmed. At the time, I had just moved into my home and home practice, so when film directors and producers all came round for a meeting, they had to sit on boxes rather than chairs. It was soon decided that I should travel out to the set to treat the actor there. I still cringe at the first phone call I got when I was busy in the clinic, with someone telling me that the BBC was sending a car to pick me up. My honest reply was that I had to go home first as I had washing on the line and a cat to feed! A chauffeur then turned up in a large, shiny car, and I was off.

I had my bear backpack on, which was full of chocolates, as well as laser and acupuncture needles. "Are you a famous chick?" I was asked by the driver. I said no and the window was raised between the front and the back of the car.

It was a quiet drive, but it was amazing to be driven just as fast backwards as forwards… I've tried this myself, and I can't do it! Quite a skill.

Once I got there, 'Darling' got my actor to have chocolate for breakfast, and I was told that if they ever had to act the part of a specialist who was totally weird and who had a crazy sense of humour, they would think of me. Needless to say, I wasn't quite sure how to take that! I had to make a TARDIS type clinic in a small caravan on site, and I hopped on set to nurture a sore neck through flying scenes (where the actor was suspended on ropes) and a death scene in a coffin (which, to tell the truth, was extremely dull to sit through).

I also attended to various mild back pains from the script writers and directors, who were in pain due to prolonged posture from standing around the set all day. This caused small muscles to get painful and the oxygen supply to get trapped in the lower spine. There was also frustration and anger at impending deadlines, causing TMS (Tension Myositis Syndrome) so there was quite a lot to keep me occupied. The good news was that the scenes continued without any delays, thanks to my snazzy techniques.

As I've mentioned, it is difficult to act comfortably when you are in pain or stiff, as body language has to be congruent with the mood and age the actor is acting. This made me think about how fit actors have to be; they have to act a certain age or fitness, and they must also mimic the natural ageing process and how we move differently. They spend a lot of time getting to the correct size and level of fitness for the part, and core work is the key to everything in terms of the quality of fluid movement. The have to perfect the way their character would walk, their purpose, their sexual orientation, their mood, everything. Posture, in particular, is key to mood – for example, if an actor is portraying a depressed person, their shoulders would be slumped forward, their voice monotone, their movements slow.

I have treated directors and actors on many occasions over the years to ensure that they are fit enough to do their jobs. Long days of hanging around on set, poor posture, and lots of stress can lead to many different types of aches and pains. Not to mention actors who are suddenly called to fall or run – that is, if the stunt man isn't doing it all. They need fitness and endurance in order for the musculoskeletal system to function without pain.

—◦◦◦—

A Striker with No Strike

One cold winter, I got a call to help a football medic and physiotherapist who had a puzzling problem: their player was repeatedly breaking down, feeling sharp tugs in his hamstrings. Of course, when you are renowned for scoring goals, this isn't very helpful, and it got to the point where he'd be too fearful to even see the game through.

So, I dutifully turned up at their hotel (we met there as the media loves to write about injuries and problems, and for sportsmen, their perceived worth can be destroyed overnight, like a race horse scenario) and it turned out that I needed to pull out my knowledge about nerves misfiring, and about muscles that feel muscle tears when there aren't any. A handful of treatments back at my office at home and he was good to go. The moral of the story here is to always check out the lumbar spine with lower limb problems, then make sure the player himself *believes* that he is fixed.

—◦◦◦—

Fit Enough to Walk

Jeff's walking holidays were everything, he told me; since early retirement from the police force, Jeff and his wife walked and climbed every mountain range they could. "My life has ended," he bitterly told me, "the Doc says my spine is collapsing and if I persist in my hobby, I could end up in a wheelchair. He may have to fuse it if I become incontinent. My wife either stays at home with me and resents it, or goes on walking trips by herself, and we drift apart due to my envy."

"Tell me about your fitness regime," I said. Jeff did no exercise for weeks at a time, then would go on long walks, carrying a rucksack full of goodies. He was obese around his stomach, and apart from the toned legs he got from walking, he had poor core and upper arm strength. His walking pattern was awful due to a limp and flat feet. His diet was reasonably healthy, he just needed some adjustments to reduce calories when not walking so much, and he needed to introduce more fresh alkalising green veggies into his food intake.

He came to my clinic to resolve the clinical spinal nerve compressions due to deep muscle contractures and ageing discs, and we made use of IMS, mobilisation of his small spinal joints, gait scan analysis, and bespoke orthotics (more on this in my next book). Importantly, post treatment he commenced his new fitness regime to enable him to walk long distances. He would get into the state to heal his body with daily morning tai chi sessions 20 minutes before breakfast, he juiced with fresh veggies most days, and in the evening he did 15 minutes of core pilates exercises on his fitball, and also used arm weights to strengthen his spine, tummy and shoulders, while watching the news.

Then, three times a week he either cycled, swam, or jogged in water to get his heart rate up. On the other days he went for a brisk walk and did breathing exercises. I taught him Tony Robbins' favourite four quick breaths in and four pants out, shouting life-affirming statements out to connect the breathing with core and mindset. Then, for stamina, he went for a long walk on a Sunday. Three months later, a jolly couple bounced into my clinic with Himalayan flags wrapped around them, and an album of photos from their latest expedition.

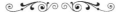

Once you've read this chapter, please go to page 251 of the appendix and complete the traffic light questionnaire for fitness again to see how you have improved.

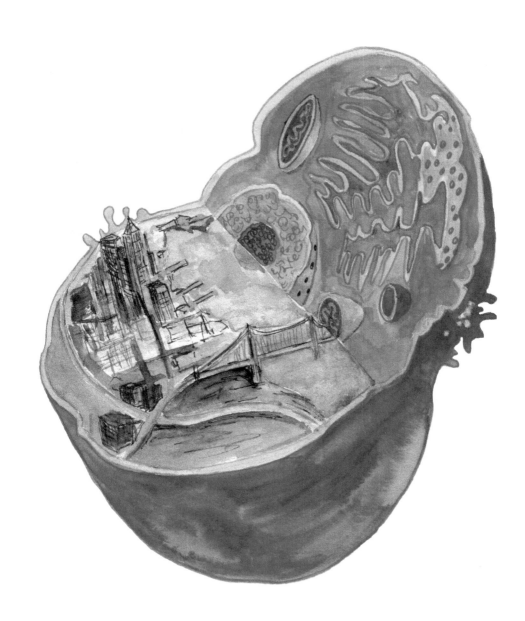

Lifestyle

Life's Most Important Treasures

Joy
in your heart,
your mind,
your soul.
Peace
with yourself
and with the universe.
Harmony.
Courage
to feel, to need,
to reach out.
Freedom
to let yourself
be bound by love.
Friendship.
Wisdom
to learn, to change,
to let go.
Acceptance
of the truth
and beauty within yourself.
Growth.
Pleasure
in all that you see,
and touch,
and do.
Happiness
with yourself
and with the world.
Love.

–Maureen Doan

Before you read this chapter, please go to page 252 of the appendix and complete the traffic light questionnaire for lifestyle.

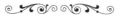

inally, we come to lifestyle, and there are several main questions here. Why do I place such importance on lifestyle? How does our lifestyle affect how healthy we are? What is it about our lifestyles that determine how long our lives will actually be?

How Lifestyle Affects Us

Personally, a recent journey of mine really made me think about lifestyle and how it can affect us, both in body and mind. It was during this year's New Year break, I was aiming to get some sun and write a bit more of my book. I thought that I'd get a lot done, away from my usual crazy life where there was hardly a single second I could have to myself. I was looking forward to it. I was looking forward to it so much, in fact, that I started writing on the plane, and I was in the middle of a sentence when my computer crashed. Luckily, I had a copy on my memory stick, so as the plane touched down on what was essentially a large rock off Africa's west coast, I remained smug in the knowledge that I could just use another computer once we'd landed.

Well, that didn't turn out so well, and what happened next made me completely rethink our modern Western lifestyle, and how many of our daily stresses are totally self-inflicted. Anyway, I arrived at the hotel and asked about their Wi-Fi and any computers they had that I could use. To my dismay, they only had one computer – a communal one in reception – and their Wi-Fi signal ended at their reception desk.

My conditioning had been so strong over the last few months – glued to my IT stuff in the car, in my office, and at my clinic, that I felt totally disorientated and lost. I realised that most of my stress came through cables and satellites and that my world revolved around answering emails and phone calls, not to mention Facebook and Twitter and reading endless online research.

Whilst I was staring miserably at my small case and my – now, pointless – IT stuff, I noticed that my tongue was as dry as toast and that my head felt fuzzy. "Cheer up, Snazzy," I told myself. All I needed was a nice cup of tea and I'd be fine. To my delight I found a kettle and a mug, but sadly no water, no tea bag, and no milk whatsoever. No tea? Suddenly my book seemed less urgent.

I queued for what seemed like forever only to be given just two small bottles of water. I was informed that due to the island seeing no rainfall for the past seven years, there was no vegetation and all water had to be imported. Therefore, they had to ration it out. On top of this, guess how tasty the food was?! I sure was missing my lovely kitchen at home, with all of its herbs, oils, spices, and fresh fruit and vegetables.

Determined to do something productive, I walked off along the coast to the nearest town in the hope of finding some paper to write on. Carrying my precious water, I took my trainers off and waded into the sea, aiming for a peaceful paddle in the glistening waves. What actually happened was that those glistening waves hurled me back onto the shore in a most undignified manner, and I remember thinking, "I'm glad I don't have to hunt my own fish", as I sat up and tried to locate my shoes on the sand. Staggering over to them, I promptly cut a hole in my mollycoddled, soft feet. Now, I was focused purely on not fainting from the pain as I hobbled three miles through uneven sand dunes, my thirst now the last thing on my mind.

Was I concerned about missing an email at this point? What do you think? As my shoulders burned in the afternoon sun, I was reminded of the physiology pyramid. At the bottom of this pyramid you had your survival issues, with thirst, hunger, and shelter being the main focus. My primitive innate responses to stress were working in the same way as they did in my normal lifestyle back in the UK, though, admittedly, to more pressingly urgent conditions necessary to survival. I thought of all the incredible survival strategies I knew about, of Brazilian monkeys that had only just been filmed in detail and how they did a much better job of surviving in the rainforest than I was currently showing on the shores of Africa. If I was on my own, with no rain and only sea water, I wondered how long it would take me to figure out how to extract the salt, and then find seeds and irrigate the land. Building a computer would be a little beyond me at that point.

At around the time of the Second World War, my own late grandfather actually installed telegraph communication cables from these islands out along the ocean beds and along the African coast. Morse code was used for early transmissions, although even back in the 1850s, these cables were laid out across the oceans, with documented information on the American Civil War being transmitted in this way. Recent evidence gathered from an Anglo Saxon find of buried treasure, near my home in the UK, discovered that the jewels and gold were sourced far away from their ultimate resting place, even from other continents. Even back then, man was travelling to collect precious metals and jewels and to create beautiful objects.

All of our lifestyle experiences today are built on the shoulders of our ancestors, and all around the world, lifestyles are as varied as nature and the environment itself. I believe that the human brain and the planet is changing and evolving all the time. They say that early man's frontal cortex evolved once he absorbed key amino acids from fish food, which allowed him to create the historic architecture and treasures that surround us in abundance in Europe.

Having a Good Foundation

If you want optimum health, you must have a good foundation and strong pillars, or it will tumble down – even if just one pillar is weak. Try sitting on a chair with three legs; you'll soon end up on the floor. It is like this with your health, and as we've seen throughout this book, each one leads into the other. You must get your head in the correct space before you do anything else, and then once you've got the correct mindset, you can change the way you eat and the way you exercise. All of these things then give you the energy and the power to change your entire lifestyle. By changing your mindset to overcome the desire for short-term gain, you can put effort and time into your healthy lifestyle planning. Make lifestyle choices through your own wisdom – don't be driven by the media.

Sadly, both the drugs industry and the food industry are primarily about making a profit, putting money before our health. Therefore, willpower is needed in order to overcome the overwhelming satisfaction of immediate, short-lived pleasurable sensations, such as eating junk food to comfort ourselves. In a stressful life, the needs and the triggers for immediate gratification are strongest. In the 1990s, a very popular low-fat diet was actually loaded with sugar to make it taste nice, and now we have seemingly 'healthy' smoothies loaded with sugar as well. We should trust these products only with intelligent questioning. After all, diabetes is a modern lifestyle area of growth, and remember – we could all do with being taller for our BMI!

How Our Behaviour Affects Our Lifestyle

When it comes to being healthy and having a good immune system, what's the big deal? Well, the way we live our lives shapes our future through our genome, conducting the orchestration of our gene pool. These include things such as social life, family, culture, network, connections, hobbies, groups, neighbours, family, love, friends, work, identity, status, environment, home, building, house, work/life balance, frequency of human touch, conversation, and daily interaction.

I once read somewhere that in terms of human touch, South America leads hands down on this. The USA is second to last, and the UK is last. What does that say about us? Add touch and hugging into your lifestyle – it's an excellent medicine, and it doesn't cost a thing.

Physical wellbeing is, in part, created or destroyed with our lifestyle. There has been a lot of scientific research carried out on this subject, with multitudes of data we can study. For example, we know from looking at retirement and multiple personalities that our career – and especially, a purposeful vocational career – has a profound effect on our health. According to a worldwide survey, 80% of people do not like their job, and a job can represent a lot in a person's life. In fact, at one of his seminars, Deepak Chopra told us that more people die on a Monday morning at 9 a.m. than at any other time. Time sickness is a real thing, and if we don't believe we have enough of it, nature tends to agree with us.

Deepak also told us of one study that looked at rules of disengagement at work. If your boss ignores you, you are likely to suffer 45% of disengagement and increased sickness, and 30% if you are criticised. If even one thing about you is praised, however, there is minus 1% disengagement. Out of this study came the importance of creating an environment where people are encouraged to discuss each other's strengths and play to them, making work life more rewarding and less disappointing.

Investigating Our Cells

I am going to take you back in time now to the moment of your creation, when you were initially a sperm and an egg, and then a cell, and then many more cells. I want you to really understand who you are, how you function and keep healthy, and how pain is a messenger to warn you when your cells are unhappy.

With the aid of scanning electron microscopes (SEM) back in the late eighties, I could literally fly through cells. This led me to thinking about atoms and how they are empty, and later on to thinking about quantum energy, and then on to finding explanations for spontaneous remissions and healing treatments. I will explore this in more detail in my next book, *The Human Garage*.

Once upon a time, a healthy, determined sperm buried itself in an egg. There was one day of rest, then you started growing, and after this, you specialised, and these very few cells can create anything. Your cells are partly shut down to only make bone, or skin, or hair. An intelligence directs the positions of your embryo cells by sacred geometry, and then chemicals start a cascade of information to direct whether your own particular cell is a stone mason or a carpenter and so on. This then specialises, and the regenerative properties diminish. As I said, our cells are positioned according to sacred geometry, something which Leonardo da Vinci knew only too well; he has a famous painting with these dimensions in (it is also the helical arrangement of DNA).

You can think of your cell as being a tiny version of you. It has a memory, a brain, and a stomach, and just like us, it has its needs. The cell membrane is the equivalent to our own brain, and it is very specific about what it lets into and out of the cell; our cells protect us, and actually control our future by determining what we can and can't do. They not only give us qualities that have been passed down through our ancestors, but they also adapt to their environment. For example, we think of cancer as being a very hereditary thing, but it isn't always so. A child with no history of cancer in their own family can develop the disease if they are adopted into a family who have all had cancer.

As you can see, cells are fascinating things. Many studies have shown that more primitive organisms can regenerate their cells, such as the salamander, and even when we are babies, we can regenerate cells in the tips of our fingers. As we grow up and our cells become more specialised, however, we lose the ability to regenerate our cells, which is why we have to look after ourselves more as we get older.

Very small things can affect our cells. When I was a third year biologist, I specialised in cellular physiology, and at Birmingham University (in the biology labs in Edgbaston) I did a very interesting study. It was one of my four final research projects, and it's one I love to bring up at posh cocktail parties. I did a study on sperm health, looking at the influence of environment on sperm, and I found that when even a very diluted detergent was used to wash the pipette (which was then left to dry before being used), it altered the lifespan of the sperm. And no, before you ask, I didn't collect the samples myself!

Another experiment I looked at was mast cells, which are key in asthma attacks. I induced a reaction, and when I sent a biochemical trigger through the cell membrane, I photographed it using scanning electron microscopy techniques. These facts meant that I could embrace pioneering technology which is new to the UK (MRT) and see its role with physiotherapy, sports injuries, and arthritis. If you are an entrepreneurial type, it is sensible to have all your ground work in place.

The Cell as the Basis for Our Environment

Anyway, let's look at a cell, which is one trillionth of you. It has a brain of its own – the membrane – and it works in a very specific way. The receptors on the surface of the cell can recognise electromagnetic signals, and it is now believed that they also include thoughts, nutrients, hormones, and chemical messengers. The nucleus is essentially the heart of every cell, and could be referred to as its control centre. If removed, the cell will die within weeks. If the membrane – the brain of the cell – is removed, then there is instant death.

Is the way we live a cleverly evolved, thought out process? Or is it simply a reflection of us – or of our cells (to be more precise)? Let's look at our homes. Why do we build them the way we do? We have doors so we can allow who we want in, and keep out who and what we don't want to enter. We give our houses rigid walls to give a skin/structure/lining, we have telephones to communicate through, and satellite dishes to receive signals. There is a road up to the house for vehicles to transport people and things right up to the doors, a warming fire for energy, a kitchen for food preparation, a dining room to eat food in, a lounge for us to sit in and observe information through a screen, and bedrooms to sleep in. Our homes are based on our cells.

On a bigger scale, we can also look at cells as being similar to the towns and cities we live in. A cell is, in fact, a tiny version of a city, and I find it fascinating that as humans, we create our world in our own vision, by making our cities as much like our own cells as possible. For example, every city has motorways to carry materials and food, much like elements passing through the membrane. Our telegraph poles and satellite dishes allow our cities to communicate, much like the gates and receptors in the membrane, as well as our nerve endings. Cities need sewers to dispose of waste, as well as building structures, like our bones and collagen. The restaurants in the city equate to our stomach, and our law, schools, and police that we rely on in cities and towns can be compared to our genes.

The cell allowed bacteria to invade billions of years ago, and it had a choice: kill it or embrace it. It chose the latter and became the powerhouse of our existence: the mitochondria. It is the guard, and if the cell turns on us, it actually self-destructs the cell, like a tiny but brave 007 agent. However, if we upset it with a poor lifestyle, it doesn't self-destruct. Cancer, for example, happens when Mr Mitochondria is angry.

Cells essentially taste – they're sensitive to the environment, and so your behaviour and what the cell experiences actually shapes your genes. The rabbit hole of genetics, if you will, controls the interplay of genes being switched off and on. Studies point time and again to lifestyle and mindset influencing genetic interplay and disease.

Tips for Changing Your Lifestyle

If you want to start changing your lifestyle right now, there are several small, simple things you can do to get you heading in the right direction. Here is a list of just some of them:

- Get a regular massage.
- Meditate daily, even if just for five minutes.
- Exercise daily, both aerobic and strengthening.
- Stretch and relax with vital Eastern exercise.
- Move with good posture.
- Set purposeful goals – both big and small – and plan how to achieve them.
- Do something nice for a stranger.

- Watch less TV.
- Study something every day.
- Communicate effectively and praise others.
- Eat moderate portions of good, nutritious food and take the time to enjoy it.
- Hydrate with good water.
- Be aware of breathing and stressful thoughts.
- Spend time with inspiring and funny people.
- Build healthy relationships.
- Explore the tantric side to sex.
- If you care, say it.
- Be passionate.
- Have a vocational job.
- Get some daily daylight.
- Give yourself an instant reward for achieving goals.
- Allocate focused family/friend time.
- Allocate focused hobby time.
- Dance a few minutes every day.
- Sing in the shower.
- Enjoy your home and work environment.
- Have plants and flowers inside where you live and work.
- Create a spiritually healthy space.
- If you are in pain/injured/arthritic, seek professional advice in both traditional and alternative medicine.
- Use my traffic lights approach to health.
- Read my next book on the Human Garage.

Making More Time

Focusing on how little time you have left can make you happier. It sounds strange, doesn't it? We have to look to the future to appreciate the present. If you have suffered pain or a loss of movement for some time – or maybe if you've had repeated episodes of sports injuries – your physical problems will have led to an ever-increasing restriction on your lifestyle, or on your inability to play your favourite sport. This starts the vicious circle of less exercise and mobility, falling fitness, and depression, which makes your pain worse or your injury more frequent. And so it goes on. All this isn't helped, of course, by your stressful lifestyle, which is often complicated by a poor diet of junk or heavily processed food. The results can be a spiralling certainty of obesity, diabetes, heart disease, cancer, and osteoarthritis to name just a few.

Does this sound like your story? Unfortunately, it is a common one. If this is you and you aren't taking any action, you are potentially heading towards an unrelenting life of pain and even premature death. If you want to commit to positive change, there is a lot of evidence to show that you can make outstanding improvements in your quality of life – and your life expectancy – simply by taking baby steps, but you must start *now*.

Women's Wellness – Getting Older the Better Way

How Ladies Can Age In a Graceful, Contented Way

We often hear the phrase, "the autumn of a woman's life," and I chose this time to discuss because it is *my* time as I write this book. This is a time to reflect on what we've achieved and who we have cared for over our life.

Sound research from a new branch of science has shown how our belief systems are embedded in our minds, much like a virus. They call this mind virus a meme. Our belief systems are embedded with cultural memes to programme us as to how a woman should behave and dress at certain ages, often with a disempowering motive. It is how we learn how to behave in the roles of a daughter, wife, mother, lover, friend, worker, and boss that will shape future generations.

My favourite time of the year in the UK is when winter is showing signs of retreating into the coolness of early spring, where the sun's energy grants us a few minutes of more light each day, gradually erasing the sleepy, hibernating days. Being aware of the role that the seasons of life play in how we feel, act, dress, and look is important as it allows us to become more powerful women. I actually feel that the seasons are akin to the four key phases of our lives.

Spring represents the first quarter of our life, when our physical bodies are growing and we are able to repair and produce cells at a fast pace. We take good health for granted, and our minds are loaded like a computer, with language and knowledge about the rules of the world, but with very little maturity to question anything. Spring is about childhood, freedom, growing, exploring, learning, growing into who we are, and falling in love. It is our adolescence.

Summer typically spans ages 20 to 40, those years demanding a multifaceted role with reasonably sound health. We ladies are running from pillar to post with studying, careers, marriage, and if we are blessed, parenting. This busy time calls for survival and giving, rather than reflection on our own lives.

The autumn of our life, from 40 to 70, brings the time when young families have flown the nest. Hormones are changing as the child bearing years recede, but this phase in our lives leads into a difficult menopause. Healing is slower, the body needs nurturing to fire it up, we have to put effort into staying physically strong and supple, and yes, exercise is needed for weight control and looking good. The face also needs careful attention to retain a youthful glow; with raw vegetables, plenty of water, supplements, and face creams, we ladies can – and do – look stunning.

The mind is key at this stage in life, as it can be when women are most successful with their careers. For example, at 62, Louise Hay launched a most successful publishing house. However, the mind – or more importantly, our cultural beliefs – can also be our worst enemy. I meet women who say, "I'm sixty; I need to slow down". If you see yourself as getting old at 60, that's exactly what you will be.

Yet, there has never been such an exciting time for this phase of our lives. Since we have been given the vote, we now stand strong, able to command very rewarding jobs. By the 1990s, women in the USA owned around 40%

of the companies, and being more people-orientated bosses, they supplied work for many.

70 onwards and we are in the winter of our life. If we have been fortunate enough to understand and experience good health and invest in it, we can now reap the rewards. Chronic illness will be less severe and painful. We may hope to die peacefully at a grand old age after a fulfilling day of good physical and mental activities.

In the winter, the greatest fear to having an active lifestyle is falling, especially when the roads and pavements are covered in ice, so this is what we will look at next.

Tips for Fall Prevention on the Ice, Especially In the Winter of Our Lives

Being a fellow biologist, I liked Heather Urquhart's advice of walking like a penguin this winter; this quirky idea has been rated as the best approach to prevent falls in the first place. Heather, who is a biologist and the manager of the penguin exhibit at the New England Aquarium, stated, 'Keep your knees loose, point your feet out slightly and extend your arms to the sides to keep your balance' (Urquhart, 2013).

Do the penguin! Can we see that catching on? Here are a few more tips for walking in the snow and ice this winter:

- Compacted ice under snow can be lethal so sensible footwear please – no stilettos in the snow, for example. You can always put stockings around slippy shoes, as my colleague Nikki Rose suggested.
- Crampons can help, or just good old fashioned walking boots.
- No running please over snow and ice.
- Careful of being merry, and if on medication, check before you leave home. If diabetic, you will get cold outside so allow for this with your calorie intake.

- If you know you have a fragile, arthritic neck, wear a thick scarf to help protect you if you slip, and support your neck with your hand if you stumble.
- Wear sunglasses to improve visibility in the glare off the snow.
- Vitamin D can help with bones losing that wonderful sun, and there is an increased risk to fracturing bones with repeated falls.
- I get my patients to use Nordic poles for extra stability, as it takes the strain off aching knee and hip joints.
- Rucksacks – rather than bags – free hands up.
- Take extra care getting in and out of cars and up and down steps.
- Clear away anything you can off footpaths, as once covered by snow, you will not see the objects.
- Dry shoes thoroughly, and wipe them on the mat before entering buildings, as slippy wet soles can be lethal.
- If clearing a path, put salt substances down to prevent ice formation.
- If frail, then get a Lifeline Personal Help Button.

If you are someone who is scared of falling and is dreading being locked away all winter, the good news is that help is at hand. Falling is a huge subject and a lot of energy and time has been put into programmes to physically and emotionally help vulnerable individuals. If you know someone heading into winter with a history of falls, it may well be worth having a thorough physiotherapy assessment to identify additional cause(s) of falls not previously known that might be addressed.

To include falls and near misses (also indicators of falls risk), it is recommended to pose the question to yourself using the following wording: "In the past month, have you had any fall, including a slip or trip in which you lost your balance and landed on the floor or ground or lower level?" (Lamb et al., 2005). If you answer yes, then go and have a physical assessment, which should include assessment of walking (gait), balance, joint range of movement, and muscle strength.

Falls and poor bone health are a major cause of disability and accidental deaths in our older population, especially in icy conditions. Research into causative factors and prevention of falls show that many of the interventions provided through physiotherapy and exercise regimes – such as tai chi – can modify the risk and help to prevent future falls. Getting help after an immobilising fall improves the chance of survival by 80% and also increases the likelihood of a return to independent living. This research also stated that clinicians have to ensure that: 'the balance training is highly challenging, individualised and progressive. Exercise should be at least twice a week and for a duration of 6 months. Walking should only be prescribed in addition to a high intensity/high dose programme.'

Training provides you with strength and stamina; giving your heart, lungs, and the rest of your cardiovascular system even a modest workout can make a difference in the way you go about enjoying life.

It is also important to consider balance and reflexes. When you were very young, you had to learn how to balance yourself, and unless you continue to use your balance under safe conditions, this vital skill diminishes. In fact, this skill has to be retaught as we age, and this is essential when it comes to ice. Balance and good reflexes help you to keep the mass of your body over your feet, which helps you to maintain your stability when moving your weight from one position to another. Regain some of the spring in your step, and then practise walking with a stronger, safer, and more fluid gait. Then do your penguin winter walk with a smile on your face!

Why is falling such an important subject? Well, falls account for 25% of hospital admissions and 40% of all nursing home admissions. Of those admitted, 40% do not return to independent living and 25% die within a year of their fall. About one third of the elder population (over the age of 65) falls badly each year, and the risk of falls increases proportionately with age and ice. At age 80, over half of individuals fall annually, and half of those discharged for fall-related hip fractures will experience another fall within six months. In fact, falls are the leading cause of death among the elderly, and 87% of all fractures in the elderly are due to falls.

So, there is a notable trend of increasing falls in the older population, and these have been recorded as being common causes for admission into hospitals. Let's reverse the trend together this winter, and stop your wobbly friends from being scared and isolated.

Learning to Drive Again

I'd like to just add a bit of a light-hearted story here regarding a patient of mine who had fallen awkwardly on ice. I had just completed a fascinating two weeks with Richard Bandler (the co-creator of NLP), and I excitedly decided to do some light trance work. My first opportunity to use hypnosis after this particular course was with a delightful lady, a retired teacher. Due to her fall, she had a smashed up arm, which had been mended with screws and nails. Although she had come a long way since her accident, she couldn't turn the ignition key to drive, and she believed that she would never be able to do this again. Confident that I could help, I told her that she would be turning that key within the hour, and she did.

The problem was, whilst I was gently hypnotising her, she was talking about the love life of a mutual friend of ours, who was seeing a tall, broad-shouldered lawyer. When I was finished, she could indeed turn the ignition key, but she later rang me up in hysterics – every time she went to put the keys in the ignition, her brain associated this action with the tall, broad-shouldered lawyer, so every time she held the key, she felt like she was holding something of his, if you get my drift! I told her I could try and change the effect so it wouldn't happen anymore, but she declined, saying that driving had never been so much fun. Her husband, however, was less than impressed. This just goes to show that you feel what you believe is there, and I don't think I've ever had anyone who's enjoyed my treatment quite so much!

Feng Shui

Feng shui your life – a powerful key to lessening a stressful lifestyle

What is feng shui? Basically, it is an understanding of the ancient art of placement, the Chinese interpretation of the world, and the study of their stars to help create sustainable agriculture and dwellings. This is also the belief that the space and objects around us directly affect the health and success of our lifestyle. In modern day, these ancient principles are accessed to create nurturing, life-enhancing, and supportive spaces in our homes, gardens, and offices.

The Chinese talk of five influencers on lifestyle: luck, destiny, feng shui, virtues, and education, and it is all about positioning ourselves within the immediate environment that best suits our purpose. For example, my team at work are most happy if their desk is where they want it, their window has a view they like, they have the correct light, the correct temperature, the correct smells, the correct space, and any plants or knick-knacks that they want to include in that space. If the design and the colours also work for them, then happiness and success is much easier to achieve.

It is fascinating to discover the early intelligent methods of determining agricultural sites and dwellings, including wind strength, river flow, soil types, predators, and more. If I were to place plants wherever I felt like it in the gardens at work or at home, with no knowledge of sunlight positioning, soil type, or the level of shade needed, I would have a lot of dead plants, and it's the same with everything else we put into our environment.

Feng shui stems from the I Ching, which are ancient scripts that interpreted universal energies, such as lifestyle, food, and health. It also involves yin and yang opposites and the need for balance. My own knowledge of feng shui is actually very shallow compared to the scholars who have spent years and years studying this vast subject. On a side note, when I had my home practice, someone did a feng shui reading for me, which resulted in having a water fountain in my office. This was great until one of patients dropped his trousers in it – I explained that it was good feng shui but he wasn't convinced.

Although it is undeniably extremely complex, I love the concept of feng shui. I understood from studying Chinese acupuncture, shiatsu, meditation, tai chi, and chi kung that it was all seamlessly interconnected. Now, feng shui embraces the five personality element types, much like the game metal, fire, earth, water, wood. Its characteristics are akin with the seasons, colours, objects, shapes, moods, desires, and abilities. Your personality trait then combines with Chinese astrology, depicting 12 compass points, each with an animal name related to the time you were born. This gives you an animal name to depict behaviour. Personally, I am a dragon – say no more.

When I had the feng shui expert at my house, I was just getting my head around everything when the lady produced a bagua – a sort of magic square likened to a cosmic computer – to see how my house would affect my health and fortune. Islamic, Hebrew, and Tibetan cultures all use these, and I saw them everywhere when I was out in the East. They combine horoscopes with numbers and locations, using the directions of North, South, East and West. You are then given a number to depict a magical template of your life.

Although this is all a long way from our Western culture, assessing a house move using this thorough method makes a lot of sense. Many times, my patients retire and move to somewhere remote, or go to the coast, or they downsize or they give up a garden. They get depressed and ill as it's not right for their personality, and in marriage you have two very different souls with diverse needs to please.

The psychological impact of our environment is our very key to happiness: do we like the country? The quiet? Remote places? Shopping? Being around people? Being around friends? Do you know yourself and the lifestyle that suits you best?

I recently had a lesson in not really knowing myself. I had worked through the whole summer, stuck inside my clinic with the sun pouring through the window. So, I made my mind up: I would have a few days in the sea and sun, and boy was I bored, and shocked that I was! Here's another interesting thing to think about. If you have them, get your dowsing rods out (mine are always on my desk). A dear friend of mine showed me how to dowse and took me through the history of the ley lines in my village, as well as the effects of them within my house and study. The geology of the earth also has a part to play with geopathic stress lines, meaning that earth disease, underwater streams, mines, railways, and roads all affect the electromagnetic flow around us. Ley lines are the acupuncture lines of the earth, as a shaman out in New Mexico explained to me. These shamans used to communicate through these, and in many cultures – including Chinese – ley lines are read to find out suitability for buildings and health. Modern day German scientists Hartmann and Curry described earth grids as force lines activated by the earth's magnetic field and the gravitational pull of the sun and moon. I have a strong ley line through my study at home which I used to treat patients in, and this same line had a history with a row of houses in the adjacent street.

Going back to my feng shui visit, I went on to be told that I had instinctively placed sounds, smells, and touchy feely, visual stuff in the right places: waterfalls, plants, candles, soft rugs, fabric, aromatherapy smells, candles, open windows, and mirrors… they were all in places to soothe the soul, and I carried forward these ideas in my current clinics. Unfortunately, I am also guilty of clutter, which I need to address. This reflects in my personality of often doing things out of duty, and of being fearful of jumping into the unknown.

Understanding Colour

This brings me onto colour. I love having time to oil paint with colours, mixing them up to create the perfect hue. Humans use colour to convey unspoken words and feelings, and we can have innate connections with certain colours, or associated memories that trigger certain feelings. In terms of painting the walls in your house, feng shui suggests that colours should be used in particular rooms: red only on an accent wall, yellow for halls and kitchens, green for bathrooms and conservatories, purple, pink, and blue for bedrooms and therapy rooms, black accent in bedrooms, orange in living rooms, dining rooms, and halls, brown for studies, and white for bathrooms and kitchens.

At school we were taught to mix three primary colours: yellow, red, and blue. However, in 1878, a German scientist by the name of E. Hering said that the eye had colour sensors that peaked at three colours: blue, green, and red, which when mixed together, made 16 million colours. He went on to say that there are three signal channels that are connected to the brain: black and white, yellow and blue, and red and green. We all have our own interpretation of colour, and scientists suggest that colour can influence our lifestyle greatly, if used intelligently.

Here are some general assumptions about the meaning of colours that we wear, paint, and decorate pottery and jewellery with, and the appropriateness of these colours to our lifestyle.

- **Reds (cherry, rose, burgundy):** give out mood tones of boldness, dynamic vitality, excitement, pain-free, prosperous, warm, strong, powerful, danger, energy.
- **Auburn:** patient, practical, stable.
- **Brown:** connecting to nature and animals, stability, comfort.
- **Chocolate:** insightful, linked to nourishing earth.
- **Bronze:** business-like, wealth, vital, fearless.
- **Amber:** relationship bonding, creative, fun.
- **Orange:** nurturing yourself, easing fear, boosting immunity and stamina, helps chest and kidney complaints, balance.
- **Tangerine:** fun and spontaneous play, creativity, confident, determined.
- **Peach:** gentleness, kindness, friendliness, helps stress get unstuck and soothes chest problems.
- **Apricot:** creative fun, fear release.
- **Gold:** clarity in decision making, knowledge and joy, abundance, healing.

- **Yellow:** sunshine, pure, detox, intellect, mental stimulus, think, aids digestion and diabetes.
- **Lemon:** innovative thoughts, outside the box.
- **White:** pure, clarity, understanding, peace, truth, surrender, faith, holiness, helps skin problems.
- **Pearl:** calms, personal integrity.
- **Brilliant white:** start again, wipe slate clean.
- **Silver:** persistence, peace, calm nerves, protect, resolve.
- **Black:** strength tester, protect, retreat, resolve, shadow self, divine wisdom, unobtrusive, inconspicuous, mystery, self-control, saying do not intrude.
- **Grey:** coping with challenging situations, alternative point of view, magnifying glass to blocked areas, willingness to comply and detach.
- **Green:** nerve settling, good for heart and liver problems, meditating, healing, feeling less ill, less trapped and less restricted.
- **Jade:** take action and make life easier.
- **Aqua:** soothe, meditate, peace.
- **Cyan:** clarity with choices and confidence in self.
- **Azure:** protection for these life changing decisions.
- **Emerald:** calms frustrations.
- **Blue**: sky, calm, vital, healing, antiseptic, helps ability to see info, aids communication, need for detachment, rest, solitude.
- **Indigo:** clarity of purpose, insomnia aid, mental emotional ease.
- **Sapphire:** healing, regenerating, soothing nerves, purifies, aids emotional pains, aids wellbeing.
- **Plum:** devotion, dedication, commitment to life's purpose, deep bonds in friendship, overcome challenges.
- **Lilac:** psychic, faith, freeing up old patterns.
- **Mauve:** gentle, soft, intuition, spiritual, aids ears and eyes.
- **Lavender:** leadership, immunity, mind, body, soul, insomnia.
- **Violet:** regenerate, aids CNS and insomnia, creative, intuitive.

Plants and Flowers Inside a Building

Recently, there have been studies to scientifically prove an improvement in health and happiness and a reduction in stress. Behavioural research at Rutgers – the State University of New Jersey – concludes a positive impact on social behaviour, feelings of life satisfaction, and happy emotions. Professor Haviland-Jones echoed these discoveries as the director of emotion lab, where he conducted a ten month study of flowers given or set down in a house (Haviland-Jones, Hale, Rosaris, Wilson, McGuire, 2005). In summary, receiving flowers resulted in immediate happiness, less overall depression, anxiety, and agitation, and improved social connections.

On the other hand, Professor Roger Ulrich looked at the impact in the workplace, finding that men generated 15% more ideas with flowers/plants present. Professor Tove Fjeld again confirmed this with an improvement in health problems associated with an indoor atmosphere. Repeated studies have confirmed that the presence of potted plants reduced BP, and improved reaction times, attendance, attentiveness, productivity, wellbeing, perception of the space, job satisfaction, and when in hospitals, post op recovery. In one experiment at an agricultural university in Norway, 59 employers were rigorously tested. Having plants in their office resulted in 255 less health problems, 30% to 40% less coughing/dry throat/hoarseness, 25% less skin dryness, and 20% to 30% less fatigue and headaches.

Similar results were found with patients and workmen having a view of plants and trees rather than a concrete wall. Imagine all this improvement in your lifestyle, just from putting plants into your workplace!

Aromatherapy, the Scent of Flowers, Incense and Dried Herbs

Did you know that the rarest aromatic flowers were offered as sacrifices to Gods? In many ancient civilisations, incense heightened the senses during magical rites and scents were aligned with magical goals. Modern day federations still promote the healing powers of aromatherapy in massage and burners, and many scents are said to have physiological effects. My home and clinics always have aromatherapy and incense vapours, and I have my flowers and herbs surrounding my house on all four sides. American Indians use it for food, medicine, perfume, and decoration. When I was learning from the shaman in New Mexico, I remember the smells of sage, cedar, and sweet grass over hot stones in a tepee, things that are used for purification rites. A few other examples are fuzzy weed, to attract love or for good hunting, fragrant bedstraw for female perfume, and columbine and blood root for men. Evening primrose is used to avoid snakes and to attract deer.

Back in 1500 C.E. ancient Hawaiians used tropical plants in rituals and secular purposes. Between 500 and 1000 C.E. Europeans and Asians brought hundreds of tropical flowers with them, scenting clothing and bedding and making massage oil. Fragrant flowers were also worn in dance and were made as offerings to their Gods. Maile is a leafed vine, which is both sacred and strongly smelling, hala a magic perfume for sex, and puklawe is an incense to allow chiefs and commoners to meet.

The ancient Sumerians and Babylonians used incense as medicine, given to them by priests to rid the body of disease bearing spirits – juniper, cedar wood, pine, cypress, and myrtle being popular. The Ancient Egyptians traded cinnamon, frankincense, myrrh, and sandalwood for gold, and jars of it were found in tombs, ready for the afterlife. Scents were used in the home, on clothes, for medicine, for religion, and for magic and cooking.

Greeks had homes that were designed to have doors which opened out onto herb and flower gardens. They crowned their sportsmen with bay leaves, and enjoyed roses, carnations, lilies, myrtle, cardamoms, marjoram, and iris. When Greece fell to Rome, they overused perfume so much for earthenware pots, body, and clothes, that they forbade private citizens to use it.

Crystals

Crystals are used by healers for specific energy problems in the body and house. Beyond this, they make pretty additions to adorn your surroundings. Personally, I have fountains and dishes full of them from my mother's crystal shop.

Space Clearing Rituals

Here are some briefly sketched out rituals I have learnt from gifted shamans from different cultures over the years. They are only rough guides, but it's always great to learn from experts. I think it's important to be reverent to the layout, sculptures, and objects in someone's home, as well as being respectful of its energy, spiritual sense, and physical presence. It tells a story about the culture and lifestyle of those that live there. For example, the energy, books, gifts of angels, Egyptian cats, shamans, feathers and so on in my study are sacred to me.

There is evidence that humans have believed in space clearing for over thousands of years, showing that they've always wanted to live within a sacred, blessed space. Making a living place feel special means clearing away not only the clutter, but also negative energies and 'atmospheres' by using disciplined rituals involving sacred objects and herbs. My friends speak of how a place makes them feel before they describe the colours, size, and design – that first feeling is the most important by far.

Carl Jung wrote about the primeval part of the subconscious mind only being able to access ancient memories by symbols not language, accessing instinctive memories from thousands of years ago, locked within our genetic coding. These days, the power of symbols is used more for purposes such as advertising. The modern day Christian bell and Bible was demonstrated by a dear belated spiritual friend when I moved into my home. They performed an exorcism ritual and a house cleansing, telling me that it was incredibly important if you were psychic and moving into another dwelling. The old order of the Rosicrucians also taught me a lot about beliefs. They were a closed sect with the likes of Pythagoras and Leonardo da Vinci being privy to sacred knowledge. I studied with them briefly a long time ago and they have many fascinating ideas, including the notion that some of the ancient pyramids were schools of learning.

Shamanic Space Clearing

In terms of shamanic space clearing, the shamans use a smudge stick – a popular one being sage, lavender, and thyme. I have an enormous and very ancient sage plant by my front door, which is starting to look very jaded. I also have a smudge stick given to me by American Indians out in New Mexico, which, at one point, successfully set off the hospital fire alarms (and I realise I am mentioning this just when I'm talking about space clearing giving you calmness and peace)! These shamans create sacred space by calling out to power animals in the four corners: East the Hawk, South the Cougar, West the Bear and North the Buffalo. When I had the honour of joining their rituals, it was very moving.

Wiccan Space Clearing

Witches who worked alone – not in a coven but in their own way – were called hedge witches, as they lived at the edge of communities, in a dwelling perhaps hidden by hedgerows. They were healers and midwives who used primarily herbal medicine. They believed that energy makes up the world (including your home and place of work) and they communicated with spirits in order to discover problems. Again, the four elements and directions were key to their rituals. Hedge witches all had their own ways, and some worked with elemental energies, the modern day equivalent of pixies and fairies. They also cleared internal sacred spaces for peoples' homes. This ritual created a calm space devoid of external negative thoughts and was done through cleansing and tidying, purifying by removing negative energies with magic, if needed, and consecrating with a blessing.

Again, the four compass directions were associated with the elementals:

- **East:** sylphs, the Air elementals.
- **South:** salamanders, the Fire elementals.
- **West:** the undines, the Water elementals.
- **North:** the gnomes, the Earth elementals.

Hedge witches used dark stones such as obsidian, onyx, and flint for magic clearing work. Incense and charcoal represented fire and air, and sprinkling salty water represented earth and water. Other items that are good for clearing work include herbs in a jar with a sharp object, a horseshoe in iron, spells, charms, amulets, and tarot cards. For protective spells in space clearing these were also common: angelica, garlic, cactus, rowan, yarrow, and salt.

I met various wiccans who chose to work alone and not join covens for fear of their jobs, and while they all had very different approaches to white magic, they were all sincere in their beliefs and desires to heal the planet and all its creatures. In the wrong hands, however, their knowledge could prove disastrous. For a quick clearing ritual, simply throw a pinch of salt clockwise at 4 corners asking to clear and clean away all that is not good.

It is sad to think that so many were tortured and murdered for their beliefs. In fact, the witchcraft act that called for it to be considered as a jailing offence only ended in Germany in the mid 50s. So many of these people who were persecuted were midwives and healers, who were simply tuned into Mother Nature.

Druid Space Clearing

Now onto Druids. There are some writings by the Romans – who exterminated a lot of them – but the lack of written evidence means there is a lot of guess work to be done. We do know some things, however, as they passed their knowledge on by telling stories, and the Anglo Saxons pushed them into Cornwall, Scotland, Wales, Brittany, and northern Spain. Now, my mother is Welsh, and I am not sure I want too many of these wild Celtic genes in my makeup; they had a disgusting habit of human sacrifice, burning groups alive in wooden crates. On a positive side, they had intellectual leaders who stood against the Romans, so it wasn't all bad. Their space clearing ritual is not one I was taught but involves sprigs of oak leaves, mistletoe, sage, pine, and incense. You'll also need candles of the colours black, brown, olive, deep yellow, or white, and then you say, "let there be peace" to the four corners and burn the twigs – carefully!

The Incas in Mexico also had – in my opinion – some savage beliefs. I watched a re-enacted game of ancient football, whereby the winners' hearts are cut open and their beating hearts offered to birds of prey to save their soul, home, and village. Luckily for me (and the players) they did not re-enact the last bit!

Reiki Clearing

As a reiki master myself, the concept of a reiki clearing is very dear to me. First, we will look at a brief history. Reiki, simply put, means universal life force energy, and it is a lovely touch healing technique. It is thought to connect to the work put together by a Japanese theology lecturer, called Mikao Usui, in the late 1800s, and he was also a high school principal and Christian minister. Asked to undertake a ten year study of the healing work of Jesus and Buddha, as well as the esoteric teachings of India, he started by exploring the life of Buddha. Born 620 B.C.E. on the Napal-Indian border, Buddha was born to a king and escaped his closeted upbringing in order to relieve pain and suffering. A lifestyle of non-attachment healing, and loving to material and living creatures on earth was taught, and it is here that we find the earliest records of reiki.

I'd like to talk a bit here about Jesus, who was known to be a great physician. When Jesus was two years old (and when Herod was killing boy children), there were three wise men who came into his life, and these were said to be Buddhists. Now, here is the controversial bit: scripts have been found saying that these wise men took Jesus and his family to Egypt and India. There was a mystical order on the Dead Sea where the Dead Sea Scrolls were said to be found. In 30 C.E., Jesus returns to Jerusalem where he escapes crucifixion (another teaching that is in direct conflict with Christian religions), and then he returns to India for 16 years, living be 120 years old. This is a much nicer ending than the one I was taught! Having gone to a Christian Church of England school and knowing the family Bible inside out, I find these ideas fascinating.

The records are a little sketchy but Mikao Usui was believed to have conducted a seven year project in the USA, where he read Sanskrit Indian and Tibetian scripts, possibly at the University in Chicago. On his return to Japan, he went to a Zen monastery, and when he died in 1926, he passed his closest controversial teachings and healings onto Chujiro Hayashi, who died in 1940. Before Hayashi died, however, he passed on the teachings to his wife, Chie Hayashi, as well as H. Takari, and there are records of their teachings in Alaska, Tokyo, and Hawaii. They taught fifty reiki masters between them, and so the lineage continues.

Modern courses have simplified the teachings to churn out reiki masters of little knowledge, compared to the early masters who dedicated their entire lives to it. Three key signs are used in the modern interpretation of reiki: Cho-Ku-Rei, meaning God is here, Sei-He-Kei, meaning key to the universe/man and God becoming one, and Hon-Sha-Ze-Sho-Nen, meaning the Buddha in me reaches out to the Buddha in you to promote enlightenment and peace.

I have studied anthropology, psychic phenomena, and ancient healing techniques for over thirty years as an aside from my day job, and my dear tutors – whom I still sit with at least once every three weeks – are all in their eighties. Before I arrive, they always create a sacred space, with candles lit and incense wafting as the door opens. The peace always feels like a big loving hug embracing you as you slip off your shoes and enter their space. Reiki work, practised in this place and with these wise souls, can make magical changes to the way someone lives their life, standing apart from religious labels. It has always been an honour to love these dear friends, and their words often echo in my head: "focus Nicky, listen and concentrate, such an undisciplined child in this art, but showing signs of finally maturing!"

The Ancient Egyptians believed in taking materialistic items and slaves with them to the afterlife, and while obviously a highly intelligent race – with knowledge of the Nile, irrigation, writing, art, and embalming – quantum physics and matter was not on their curriculum. Burial sites and preparing for the afterlife coloured their lifestyle.

Angelic Space Clearing

I was shown something called 'angelic reiki' within my reiki training, and the concept of angels comes from Judeo-Christian tradition, in which they protect and guide humans. Angels are mentioned in – and predate – the Bible, and I have a lovely set of angel cards that help me remember their names. Each has a colour of a candle and a strong purpose or calling for specific problems.

Here are just a handful of my favourites:

- Michael: East.
- Raphael: West.
- Gabriel: North.
- Uriel: South.

If this type of clearing resonates with you, please see the appendix for a longer list of angels.

Zen Buddhism

Zen Buddhism looks at drawing attention to a defined area by using simple surfaces and textures in an uncluttered way, and by being aware of the space around us. Zen has its roots in China and was adopted by Japan in the 12th Century. It is identified within Buddhism, and it is used by my learned pain professor out in Canada.

What is the sound of one hand clapping? Nirvana is all about attaining peace, so a Zen dwelling is simple, quiet, and still, and a sandalwood smell, a gong, and a low simple table depict a Zen clearing ritual. I was taught chanting, and breathing is an important part of this. For example, take four deep breaths and then chant 'om' while kneeling with hands in a prayer position and eyes closed. When I learnt this, we did 12 repetitions of these chants and then bowed to the east, imagining the prayer casting ripples of light out to infinity. When I studied shiatsu, creating a sacred space prior to our classes – with prayer and chanting – was a clever way for us all to calm down and focus on working with the energy within meridian lines.

An Eastern Approach to Lifestyle

Since ancient times, health has always encompassed lifestyle: how we lived our lives, where we lived, how we prayed, and how we worked. Indian, Chinese, and Tibetan Buddhism – as well as Arabic and Islamic influences – all combined lifestyle, diet, mind, movement, and disease when looking at health.

Chinese Medicine

Chinese medicine dates back some four thousand years, where as well as acupuncture, at least 300 herbs were prescribed. Japan came to learn of this medicine in 5 C.E., calling their version 'kampo'. As we know from feng shui, lifestyle is all seemingly interwoven in their approach to health. Tibetan medicine from the 7th Century is a synthesis of Chinese, Indian, and Arabic techniques, and this system looks at imbalances you are born with in their interpretation of three humors: wind (movement and breath), bile (digestion, complexion, and temperature), and phlegm (sleep, joint movement, and the elasticity of the skin). They place a great importance on a disciplined mind and talk of three poisons: attachment, aversion, and confusion. They place importance on the weather, living space, environment, soil and diet, conduct in life, and so on.

They also combine medicine with prayer and rituals and see it as one practice; many doctors are monks and vice versa. They diagnose – not unlike the Chinese – by using meridian lines, pulse, tongue, and (more differently) urine. Urine analysis came from the Persians (medieval European medicine) and was exceptionally well developed. Counselling

– about lifestyle, behaviour and diet – was combined with prayer, herbs, acupuncture, and massage.

Arabic/Islamic Medicine

Arabic/Islamic medicine in the 7th Century came about when they adopted Greco-Roman traditions. As far back as 130-200 C.E., Galen – a Greek physician – studied anatomy and drugs. He was followed by Ibn Sina, a 10th Century Persian physician, who developed a system of botanical medicines and dietetics for mind, body, and soul medicine. The Muslims, who invaded India in the 11th Century, brought this knowledge and their drugs with them. Again, this was a holistic approach looking at lifestyle/climate, food and drink, physical activity, sleep, emotions, excretion/urine, and pulse diagnosis. The concepts they were concerned with were four elements, nine temperaments, and four humors: blood, phlegm, and yellow and black bile (from the Greek influence). Prayers were prescribed, along with herbs and dietary advice, and interestingly, steam and hydrotherapy. Hospitals were being built throughout the Islamic world as early as the 8th century.

Ayurvedic Medicine

Ayurvedic medicine is said to be the oldest and most completed medical system, and it has been documented from 3,000 B.C.E. The ancient holy scriptures of Vedas and Samhitas even talk of surgery and acupressure. Here, the human body is seen as part of the universe. In brief, it is divided into five elements: ether, air, fire, water, and earth relating to hearing, touch, sight, taste, and smell. Prana is life force energy, like chi in Chinese. The physical is controlled by three forces: Pitta (heat and energy), which is linked to the sun and controls digestion and biochemistry, Kapha (water and tides), which is linked to the moon, fluid and metabolism, and Vata, which is linked to the wind and controls the nervous system and movement. Holistic treatment includes meditation, diet, yoga, exercise, posture, sleep, and lifestyle issues, as well as herbs and medicines (Shealy, 2011).

Knowing your body type is another key to lifestyle choices. Fascinatingly, Ayurvedic medicine explains the type of lifestyle most suited to your body type in order to give you the best health (Chopra, 2010). It also echoes some of the Western ecto, endo, and meso that I talked about in the fitness chapter, but in more detail. Your body type favours certain types of diet, exercise, and daily activities, as well as the time for doing them, and it also makes being healthy less painful – if you understand what is easier for you.

Ayurvedic doctors teach balanced breathing called Pranayama, where they gently breathe through one nostril and then the other. The idea is to balance the left and right brain activity and soothe it before meditating (Chopra, 2009).

Modern day therapies are covered in my next book, *The Human Garage*.

Tantric Sex

Here's an interesting aspect deeply imbedded in Ayurvedic beliefs: that tantric sex is the key to peaceful, spiritual, loving sex. The origins of tantra have been traced back five thousand years, and its roots were originally in India (Hinduism), then Tibet, China, Nepal, Japan, and south-eastern Asia. Tantric symbols are found in Stone Age caves, ancient Egyptian, Hebrew and Greek mystical writings, and in ancient Arabic love songs. Sadly, when the Muslims invaded India in the 13th century, they slaughtered many tantrists and destroyed many ancient manuscripts. Even recently, the tantric practice was attacked in Tibet.

Tantra shares a lot with Taoism, an ancient Chinese philosophy. Wayne Dyer's books on Taoism helped me greatly to understand the way to achieve a state of oneness with the universe, and to achieve a state of tranquillity and harmony leading to health. Just a note here: good sex requires a fit, supple body. Body awareness is very healthy, and yoga is said to be a great way to prepare for tantric sex.

Going back to tantric sex in its truest form involves complex rituals to lovemaking, and it is believed to reduce stress as well as having healing benefits. The belief is in accepting responsibility for your own sexual pleasure and not blaming your partner, and the key to sexual bliss is finding the current – the sexual energy in yourself and your partner. An understanding of the chakras and flow of chi is important, and yoga, meditation, dance, music, and sex are all said to unblock these.

For the main chakras and their meanings, look back to the mindset chapter.

The aim of lovemaking is to awaken the Kundalini, a dormant serpent capable of either great healing or destruction, which resides in the base chakra and rises up. In Hindu tradition, the Shakti (female) and Shiva (male) originally united to form the universe, and yin and yang symbolise that union, sharing ching, which is sexual energy.

Kinesiology

Kinesiology (the study of the mechanics of body movements) is an alternative way to look at our beliefs if we feel stressed; taking practical steps to change unhealthy core beliefs can change the way you lead your life, and can also lead you to healthier, life changing mantras.

Often we are blind to our true beliefs, and there is an interesting test I have seen my sports therapist carry out. They tell me it is kinesiology, and the aim is to look at the congruency between thoughts and strength. It is all about how, if the subconscious doesn't like something, then the muscle strength noticeably weakens. In her book *Conscious Medicine*, Gill Edwards describes an arm test which my colleague Dean uses at the practice (Edwards 2010).

This exercise is for when someone shows an aversion to something, and you can try it out at home, working with a partner. Hold out your arm parallel to the floor, and get your partner to stand to one side, holding your shoulder lightly while asking the arm to stay strong. Get your partner to ask a question, making sure they avoid eye contact. Then feel the response, looking for a brief strong bounce. If you are working on your own, you could do the sway test – for example, forward for yes, backward for no. When you find a key problem, you will need to employ NLP techniques in order to anchor a new belief.

Ancient and Modern Knowledge of Treating Pain

Acupuncture is a very interesting area of alternative healing. Acupuncture points have been known for thousands of years, and were called caves. To the Chinese, they are control centres in the messaging system, meridians being channels of communication which carry chi. At acupuncture points, chi can be changed and diseases can be treated. Excitingly, it has only recently been discovered that these points may be directly over undifferentiated stem cells – cells that can regenerate. In fact, an ancient European lady was recently excavated showing these acupuncture points on her body, from over three thousand years ago. How did they know about this all those years ago? My Mayan shaman said that they also used thorns in these points thousands of years ago in Mexico, which is just fascinating.

When I was out training to lecture in pain, I discovered that in Korean hospitals, they blended Eastern and Western medicine, looking at both old and new techniques. In China, they were more secretive with their knowledge of acupuncture and pain points, and I have to say, I didn't like it when they used acupuncture with mild sedation for operations. Years ago, before metal was mined, they simply used sharp bones for needles.

Over the years, ancient knowledge has been destroyed, which is extremely sad – all of that intelligence, all of that information, just gone. Whilst I sat in a Red Indian tepee, I was told of how the storytellers were murdered, and the old medicine knowledge lost. While out in New Mexico, I did manage to find some fascinating books, but compared to what there once was, there is now so little knowledge left to access.

Soul Midwifery

I feel that this is a fitting place to talk about the subject of soul midwifery. Having sat in spiritual circles for thirty years, worked on many projects with close psychic friends, and also having undergone reiki training for over twenty years, I can guide your thoughts on this matter with authority. This is a deeply personal and emotional subject and no one should – or could – tell you what is your truth and your plan. I will just add that by having a plan as to where, how, and with whom you wish to end your days, you can give this to relatives, who will find it very helpful. Being a soul midwife is as much about being there for the dying as it is about being there for the friends and relatives.

Reiki, for example, teaches us that we all have an aura, an electromagnetic field that stretches some ten feet around us. The etheric is the part of our aura that is close to the skin, which expands with chi during sleep, and the rest is a wider energetic field. Gifted healers – like my dear friends – say that the colours and shapes in this field change in stages as someone is dying; they tell me that as the dying person weakens, the etheric body thickens and charges up with the outpouring of chi from the chakra. We are forever hearing of a surge in energy and communication prior to death, and the energetic aura fades as the soul goes in and out of the body, almost at times like leaving a pilot light on.

Let me give you a gentle introduction to how you can help a dying friend. Before entering the room, take some deep breaths and leave your day, your worries, and your personal aches and pains behind. Check your emotions and steady yourself. Make sure that you ground yourself, and that you feel balanced; imagine your feet are deep tree roots. Place one hand on your heart and then place your hands gently on your friend, connecting with the felt sense. If you are familiar with healing, gently place your hands on key chakra points – being mindful of a gentle touch only – and send thoughts of unconditional love to heal or guide the soul on its journey, for that individual's greater good.

This was a very powerful lesson learnt very recently with my friend, June. Ken, June, Lesley and I had practised the dying visualisation on many occasions, in order to ease the soul out and leave the spirit essence and body to die. It felt very different when it was one of us who was dying for real, however. June was repeatedly on the cusp of dying, all her energy levels on the pilot setting and her organs shutting down, and yet her soul would not leave. Her soul wanted to feel unconditional love and had a purpose to still make a difference in people's lives. I took photos as her eyes, skin, and limbs deteriorated, but then a voice and strength came surging through, beyond any medical explanation. This is not possible when cells reach a crisis point – however, up until this point, it is possible. Furthermore, pain, fear, lack of purpose, lack of love, and grief can kill even healthy cells.

Aromatherapy for the dying is a nice art, and can help them relax. Try bergamot, chamomile, frankincense, marjoram, sandalwood, lavender, neroli, cypress, elemi, helichrysum, myrrh, palo santo, petitgrain, ravensara, rose, or spikenard.

Spikenard is an ancient sacred oil said to have been used by Mary Magdalene to anoint Jesus at the last supper. I use frankincense in this way with reiki, past life regression, and trance work to times of trauma in order to reinstate healing. Another favourite of mine is rose, and while it is not always easy to get the right smell, it is good for grief. Petitgrain eases negative thoughts, while lavender helps sleep. Elemi (which, unfortunately, I have run out of) was brought to me from a patient from Arabia, and burning it in an oil burner gives a spiritual, peaceful air. Some people like to use one of these key oils to anoint with: sandalwood, amber, rose, or spikenard. Angelica can be used if more awareness is asked for, and rosemary can be used to help the transition for a less experienced soul. Using your thumb, simply place a spot of oil on the forehead, heart and feet with words of gratitude for that person's existence.

I also lit various coloured candles for June. I have discussed colour in depth, so I pause only to share that I will have pinks, purples, and black to settle, and oranges and reds to stimulate activity. Also, flowers and throws all add emotional hues. Angels, crystals, tarot cards, sentimental stuff… fetch it all and let them hold, touch, and feel all the sentiments that go with these objects. Once we got June out of hospital and back to her healing room at home – although still in a hospital bed, due to deep pressure sores and no muscles – she was once again surrounded by all her treasured belongings and she grew in strength. When June's heart was struggling to beat and her kidneys were failing, her lungs fought to get enough oxygen in. I matched her breathing with mine, and then used visualisations of white light going through my hands into her chest to let air in. We had windows open and a fan going, and with a tie she could control the fan, even if breathing was hard.

Although it can be a difficult thing to even think of, it can be helpful to write down a brief outline of what you want your funeral to be like, including the music and the flowers you want, as well as where you want your ashes (or grave) to be, and of course, what you want in your will.

Three of my grandparents died middle aged, and my mother's mother had this lovely piece of prose which she chose to put on her tombstone:

'So many Gods
So many Creeds
So many paths that wind and wind
Whilst just the act of being kind is all this sad world needs.
Ella Wheeler Wilcox 1850 to 1919'

When an Angel Saved My Life, And Music Saved My Arm

One day, a frail, middle-aged man named John came to see me, his arm held limply at his side like he'd had a stroke. He had a somewhat tragic – though peaceful – look to him. He clearly struggled to use this arm, and he explained to me that due to an injury, the shoulder joint had been replaced. Much like a stroke patient, he completely ignored his right arm, as if it had no purpose for him whatsoever – as if it didn't even exist. It is true that the brain ruthlessly ignores weakened parts of the body.

When we did his health questionnaire, his fitness was red, his lifestyle was red (due to the stress of his injury and the business lost because of it), his diet was green, and his mindset was amber – he had an excellent relationship with his wife, he had strong, spiritual beliefs about destiny, but his business was stressful. He ran his own hair salon, and desperately needed the use of his arm so he could cut his clients' hair. Because of the stress of running his own business, his lifestyle was suffering.

He needed to have better use of his arm, and he needed more sleep and less pain. Physically, his shoulder was badly traumatised, and I intuitively sensed a brutal attack. When I asked, he explained that as his attacker was attempting to crack open his head, a piece of rock pierced through his shoulder. At this point, he sensed a divine presence and the attacker fled, which explained the lack of bitterness that is usually embedded in the mind and the body after this type of trauma. By the grace of God, John had survived.

Psychologically, there was a disconnect between the nerves in his neck and the muscles in his arm, and I worked on this with specific frequencies through acupuncture needles. When it came to function, however, the brain still refused to play.

Music was the final connection, and through using the keyboard, the mind remembered how the arm was supposed to move; his love of music – and the emotional triggers within it – overcame that final block. Although not perfect, the arm has now been transformed from a useless limb into one that can serve him again. This is due to his tremendous spirit.

There are some powerful lessons here. For many of us, this type of attack would lead us to be resigned to the fate of a useless arm, but for John, his inner strength and determination carried him through and made him seek a solution. In looking for help to deal with his stressful lifestyle, he found himself in a much better place – one where he could heal.

———⊶∘⊷———

Another Lady Walks In My Shoes

Laughter echoed around my stairwell as a slim, lively lady with flaming red hair limped up my stairs. Her name was Margaret, and she was distraught. "I can't walk, my feet are sore. I have wedges under my shoes to protect my toe joints. You are my last resort. No one can help me walk, but I need to take a step forward."

I couldn't help but smile to myself; when my patients use that particular metaphor, I know that they're ready to make a change. On her health questionnaire, her diet was green, her mindset was amber, but her fitness was amber to red, due to the way she walked. Her lifestyle was worst of all – red, due to the stressful nature of her job as a police woman. As she spoke, it was as if a shadow crossed her face at times, and generally, she described herself as getting 'out of puff' easily, so her heart could have become an issue.

Step One was to get a gait scan analysis to analyse the pressure patterns generated through the soles of the feet, to see what we could replace the wedges with, and to remove the rocks.

Step Two involved a physical foot assessment, looking at the badly inflamed joints and nerves, as well as Morton's neuroma, where little nerve endings between the toes get rotated.

Step Three was to give her a pain treatment that linked the spinal nerves to the nerves in the feet, in order to help communication between the two, and she was also given MRT for her arthritis. Even though she'd had excellent treatments, however, she still wasn't walking properly.

So, we looked into her mind, and I felt an overwhelming sadness, as if someone else was overshadowing her. I gently placed her in a light trance and asked her to allow me into her pain. Almost immediately, I became aware of a larger lady with wild hair, a floppy velvet hat, and matching sandals. She was dancing and overshadowing this lady.

I asked Margaret if she had got a hat to match her sandals, and she replied with, "No, the violet colour is impossible to match, and it's my late best friend's son's wedding next week. We were inseparable. When we were last dancing together, she collapsed and died. She left me behind. I've dyed my hair the same colour as hers, to remind me of all the fun we had together." Here was when I found out about the psychological angle of her case, and it all became clear to me. She was grieving for her best friend so much that she'd actually started to take on aspects of her, almost as if she was trying to become her. She was making a connection between her emotional pain and her physical pain, and her grief had interwoven with her immune system, had interfered with it, even. The guilt that she could still dance – while her friend had died – was perhaps stopping her from healing, and the stress of her job and the terrible things she had to see, day in and day out, wasn't helping. Her lifestyle was as much of a problem as the memory of how her friend died.

Gently, she was able to bridge the subconscious with the conscious and control the pain, as she now understood how the pain was cascading into her life and controlling her body. She has not completely let go as of yet, but it is so much better than it was before. The lesson here is to understand the effect of grief on the immune system, as well as how the mind works in these situations. Margaret now sees the link, and rather than trying to simply treat the outcome with drugs and surgery, we could stop the cascade of biochemistry from occurring any further.

Now, every time the grieving pain hits her, she quickly tells herself a funny, happy memory. Again, we can see just what the human mind is capable of, and in changing her mindset, she was able to change her lifestyle – from one of stress, to one where she could cope with the difficulties of her chosen career.

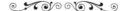

Once you've read this chapter, please go to page 252 of the appendix and complete the traffic light questionnaire for lifestyle again to see how you have improved.

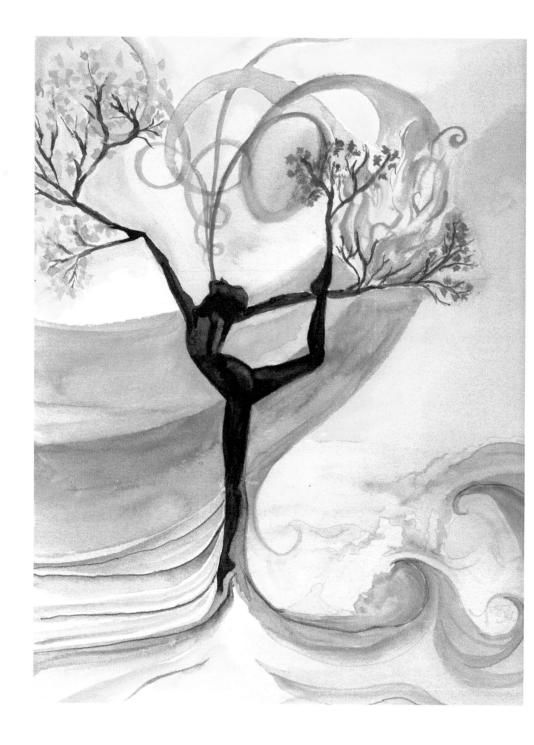

Summary

I expect to pass this way but once;
any good therefore that I can do,
or any kindness that I can show to
any fellow creature, let me do it now.
Let me not defer or neglect it,
for I shall not pass this way again.

– *Etienne de Grellet*

S o, you've read the book and hopefully you feel like you know more about pain – about where it comes from, why it occurs, and what you can do about it to give yourself a longer, happier life. Here is a brief summary of what we can do to help ourselves when we experience pain:

- **Have a massage**: nice sensations travel seven times faster than pain impulses, and this can help to block the gating mechanism.

- **Sleep**: a lot of repair work and healing takes place during this time. Some people reach the REM (Rapid Eye Movement) stage faster than others, and the time needed for adequate sleep varies partly because of this. The formation of serotonin and melatonin – 'sleep soup', if you will – is partly down to genes, and partly down to lifestyle. Amino acids, nutrients, exercise, and mindset all play a role. If you're having trouble sleeping, try a warm bath with alkaline salts and aromatherapy (especially lavender), as this will help you to relax.

- **Acupuncture**: this raises happy, pain relieving juices, serotonin, opioids, and endorphin levels, and also blocks pain at the gate.

- **Nutritious food and supplements**: the correct food products are required to make amino acids, which are essential for pain killing hormones. Minerals and anti-oxidants all reduce inflammation and boost the immune system, while too many carbs/sugars metabolise into pain products – reducing the calories reduces the pain. Less obesity: less pain. It's as simple as that.

- **Reiki and meditation**: these activities change our brain wave frequency and biochemistry. New research suggests that our state of mind has an impact on DNA transcription and chronic pain, and therefore self-healing methods like these can focus the subconscious mind on reducing both stress and pain. Reducing stress levels reduces pain and increases longevity.

- **Look at your lifestyle:** you need to view your life as if it were an activity school timetable. This will help to bring awareness to your moods. You need to look at regulating your levels of stressful or fearful activity and boost the time you spend on positive, inspiring, and emotional activities. Be honest about how you spend your time.

- **Natural biorhythms:** you need to understand these in order to make the best of your time when you're awake. When are you most alert in the day? When are you irritable, tired, or relaxed? Is there a useful pattern? During which time period are you most productive and less stressed, and does this fit with the activities you do at this time?

- **Exercise:** taking part in regular exercise boosts your endorphin levels, improves your metabolism, and helps to reduce obesity – fat cells store toxins and therefore enhance pain. Many studies prove that correct exercise significantly reduces painful chronic illness and mortality. The basic message here is: get moving!

- **Correct posture:** sitting and working correctly, as well as walking correctly, takes pain away from the small, tired muscles, ligaments, and spinal discs and gives it back to the larger, stronger supporting muscles.

- **TENS:** this stands for Transcutaneous Electrical Nerve Stimulation, and it comes in a portable hand-held device which was pioneered by a famous neuro-surgeon, Mr Norman Shealy. This medically-endorsed instrument sends frequencies – of 2HZ to 150HZ – through the sensory nerves in order to block the pain gate and boost happy biochemistry, such as serotonin, endorphins, and opioids, to kill pain, reduce depression, and help sleep. The TENS electrodes can be placed along a nerve root and onto a painful point, or onto specific acupuncture points. With the guidance of a professional, the use of a TENS machine can significantly boost the effects of pain treatment.

- **Hypnosis:** this is a fascinating and controversial subject which can significantly reduce pain when carried out by an experienced therapist. People have even had surgery whilst under hypnosis (when they are 'mesmerised'). Medical recordings were made on this technique in The Lancet journal way back in the 1830s, so it is not a new method at all. Autogenic awareness, linked with postural exercise, is great for flooding the gate with movement and positive reinforcement whilst in a trance state (and therefore in the theta brain wave mode).

- **Water:** chronic dehydration is the root cause of many painful degenerative diseases, as well as depression, excess body weight, allergies, and premature ageing. Water is medicine, and we need to be making sure that we get enough of it.

- **Breathing:** one simple conscious breath can close the pain gate, as shifting the breathing can turn on the calm parasympathetic branch of the nervous system. Endorphins help balance out the fight/flight pain impulses, and they also shift the brain frequency from beta (which accompanies the hurt if in pain) to the more calming alpha frequency. There are so many ways to breathe: calm, four-square, and circular are just a few examples.

- **Laughter:** fifteen minutes a day improves both your mood and your immunity.

I hope you try at least some of these techniques, and I hope that this book has helped you to start aiming for a healthier, happier life.

Pain relief is such a huge part of *my* life, and it is great to see pain relief knowledge being shared in the most unusual places. For example, I have a love for the National Trust and enjoy nothing better on a cool day than going and exploring some of our magnificent heritage sites. Hence, I ran a course about pain from the Shugborough Estate, as it's close to my clinic, and I used to sell Lord Lichfield's photography books in the little shop there as a teenager – so it's always been close to my heart.

My friend Professor Gunn enjoys art and culture too, and his wife, Peggy, is an excellent artist, so I thought I'd involve them in one of my courses. By this point, I'd spent years working in hospitals, and I figured that visiting different venues would be much more fun. I dragged treatment couches up flights of stairs, boxes of needles, lasers… all the equipment you need for testing one's back. One doctor – a delightful colleague and friend of the professor, and who was then working on reversing paralysis and pain – came over from France, and I was glad to see him trundle up in his 4x4 with cases of delicious champagne. I also flew Professor Gunn over from Vancouver, giving his then wonderful teaching centre over there a donation from my course. I frequented this facility a lot over the years, but sadly it has now closed with Professor Gunn's retirement, although his work still lives on: it has been reborn in Canadian sports medicine facilities at the University of British Columbia, which is great news.

Anyway, with a couple of dear friends (Steve and Laura, both of whom assisted with the practicals), we trained up a team of inspired physiotherapists and doctors who went on to do their internships at my home clinic, as well as working in UK NHS hospitals. This was before the government deemed that short, crisp discussions on exercise and drugs were the way forward, and my work lay buried… until now…

A newspaper headline in November 2014 in the Daily Express announced: 'How You Can Add Years To Your Life'. The article presented recent research from the Lancet (a medical journal) to back up previously anecdotal evidence, and basically said that having a sense of purpose as you get older helps you live a longer, healthier life. This was also echoed in Viktor E. Frankl's book, *Man's Search For Meaning* (Rider & Co, 2008), about how man's sense of dignity and purpose was cruelly stripped from him until death, and how hanging on to a purposeful mission actually extends lives.

I am currently living out that experience with my dearest friend and healing guru, whereby her sense of purpose in healing and soothing suffering is keeping her here in peace and gratitude, with a body that is in organ failure. In the newspaper article mentioned above, Professor Andrew Steptoe (director of the University College London institute of epidemiology and health) stated, 'healthy lifestyle is important, as are relationships with family and friends and finding things to do that have a sense of purpose.' He then goes on to say that people over sixty-five who have a sense of purpose are almost a third less likely to die in the next 8.5 years.

It warmed my heart to hear that The Richmond Group (which includes ten charities, including the British Heart Foundation, Breakthrough Breast Cancer, and Macmillan Cancer Support) is calling for the government, the NHS, public services, private sector, charities, and patients to work together to meet world health organisation goals of reducing preventable deaths by 5% by 2025. This requires 2.6 million people to give up smoking, 1.3 million to do more activity, 10 million to eat less salt, and 430,000 to consume less harmful levels of alcohol. At last, prevention is being given an ear.

Simon Gillespie, the chief executive of the British Heart Foundation, stated that 10,000 people die unnecessarily from heart disease, and Chris Askew, the chief executive of Breakthrough Breast Cancer, stated that breast cancer and many other diseases have common lifestyle risk factors.

The Lancet medical journal published results stating that out of 9,000 English people of an average age of sixty-five, after 8.5 years, the 9% in the highest wellbeing category had died, compared to 29% in the lowest category. Full results showed that you are 30% less likely to die if you have a high sense of wellbeing and lead a purposeful life. I've also heard that people on the UK poverty line are likely to lose twelve years of their life compared to the wealthy, which is just shocking. Other research published in The Lancet suggests ageing well has to be a global priority, and it warns health systems that we have to find ways to address problems facing an ageing population burdened by painful and stressful chronic disease.

The Office for National Statistics tells us that nearly 1 in 4 deaths – that's 100,000 per year – are potentially avoidable. That's an incredible amount, no matter what these 'avoidable' causes are. Luckily, the department of health are saying they would like to lead the world in reducing premature mortality, which is heart-warming news. This excites me as it echoes the sentiments of this book, and if you understand and embrace the knowledge within these pages, your life will be healthier, longer, less painful, and more purposeful.

So, what about my own purposeful life? What life plan did I write? My vocational core purpose was to deliver the knowledge necessary to transform lives into healthier ones, and to act as a catalyst for people to take action, as there is no power in knowledge that is not acted upon. Also, to travel internationally to achieve this, glean knowledge from gurus, and to teach not only practitioners around the world, but large audiences of the general public, as well as small groups fired up to help others make that shift. To write articles, to use the media, internet, radio, and the TV, and to work alongside celebrities skilled in transmitting information. As I sometimes present at the Z Factor using puppets to act out case studies, I would also like the opportunity to go into schools in the future, and help both parents and children understand that in order to be effective, a healthy life has to be lived from an early age. This helps to nurture sustainability.

My second key purpose was to design a clinic/clinics with treatments that embraced ancient healing knowledge along with Eastern and Western modern day medical knowledge, as well as using quantum physics applied to cutting edge technology, with a synergistic recipe to regrow cells and kill pain. To actually carry out these treatments over at least a decade, and to train up the team, evolving and fine-tuning revolutionary treatments.

I remember as a young child drawing pictures of cupboards in shops that were full of limbs – my idea was that people could replace the tired, worn out, painful ones with healthy new ones! In my story, I wanted to be part of that creation one day.

My third purpose is to teach colleagues (outside of my clinics) all these techniques I've learnt, absorbed, and honed over thirty years, to distil back into universities. This will help with my fourth endeavour, which is to get GPs, physiotherapists, health coaches, and healers to work together to help people with chronic health and mental problems.

The first purpose is wrapped up inside this book, and how I achieved the second, third and fourth ones are explored in my next book, *The Human Garage*. The spiritual coach within me shares my fifth emotional key purpose, which is my psychic awareness, my healing gifts, and the responsibility I feel I have to the guardianship of this planet. This will be covered in my third book.

Lastly, if you haven't already done so, I want you to write your life plan. After all, I think most of us have a unique calling or a purpose or two hidden away for a rainy day. Recently, with my best friend's life slipping away, I have had a rethink of my own life, looking at my frustrations about doing mundane things, such as when I have urgent deadlines always biting at my heels. I thought of how I wasted so much time having to learn about things that didn't interest me, for the sake of the businesses and helping other people. I would look at my life plan and scream out, "How will this be possible when I have all these responsibilities and duties to carry out?"

Over the last couple of decades, whenever I finished my clinical list – at around 8 p.m. – I would look longingly at my study, knowing that I wanted to write my first book. Then, life just got in the way. You know what I mean – I'm sure it happens to you too – and the draft sat there for years, just gathering dust. So, I'd then go off to do some simple building work, some painting, clear up rubble, maintain buildings, paths and gardens, do laundry, cooking, cleaning… all the usual things that take up time in your life, especially when living in a destroyed house with constant building projects going on at both the clinic and in my home. Frankly, it did my head in.

So, I continued for many years in this way, covering long lists of patients, writing endless letters, and dealing with thankless admin tasks that got dumped on my desk. Jumping on planes to go to the other side of the world for a few days to get just one piece of hopefully useful information, standing up in front of audiences and speaking to them without any prior knowledge that I would be asked to do so. Staying up, studying at stupid hours, working stupid long days, giving up years of writing and presenting and seeing friends and family – as well as giving up opportunities for exciting travel – to stay put and work on the business and treat long lists of patients to fund the clinic and the technology, when my heart was crying out to achieve my life's purpose faster.

As Jane Noble Knight said in her book, *The Inspiring Journeys of Women Entrepreneurs* (Noble Knight Publishing, 2013), I realise now that I was simply achieving it in the only way I could. "You can't connect the dots looking forward, you can only connect them looking backwards," said Steve Jobs, in his Stanford commencement address, June 2005.

I am also so thankful to those gifted souls who I've met along the way, who are brave enough to stick their necks out to make a difference, and who at times made their soul's purpose greater than their own needs. These people gave me the courage to keep going during the times when it felt like the universe was conspiring against me. I know now that the universe was simply equipping me with all the tools necessary to achieve my goals.

Jane Noble Knight summed this up in truly inspirational words: 'the world needs heart and soul centred authentic entrepreneurs, people living from their passion, behaving ethically, enjoying balanced lives, building communities, leaving legacies and feeling fulfilled. Together let's live a healthier, happier, more purposeful life.'

Acknowledgements

Thank you to my parents, for supporting me through endless education and two degrees, for buying and reading me books since an early age, and for understanding about my endless craving for knowledge.

To my brothers, Jez and Rich, and my sisters-in-law, Sara and Claire, for accepting the crazy hours I work.

To my husband, for encouraging me to become a world expert in pain relief.

June Brown, Ken Douglas, and Lesley Wilkins, thank you for your creative ideas about healing, my dear old friends. God bless you for being ears to my true self, my counsellors, and teachers of the ancient healing and psychic arts.

To my dear old friend and author, Barbara, for her words of inspiring encouragement.

To Ivan, for giving me business advice, looking after my Norfolk home, and listening to my ramblings over the years.

To my friends within the clinics, who were working away to enable me to take the time out to write my books.

My clinical team: Pam Cartwright, Dean Attwood, Katherine Kerr, David Palin, David Pinnington, Andy Pyatt, Vinod Kathuria, and Nikki Rose, all of whom implement my traffic light approach and put my patients through their paces.

Thank you to Vinod, for taking time away from surgery to fly out to Germany, meet with the MRT scientists, and to help me make the decision to bring MRT to the UK, with the help of Cell Regeneration in Stamford.

Pam, your knowledge about nutrition is amazing. Thank you TEAM for looking after 9,000 patients and helping to give them a healthier, happier, more active life.

My administration and management team: Alan Cramphorn, my husband and my finance and marketing director, for his many hours spent beavering away on projects, data, stats and finance, for implementing finance and IT systems, for easy patient note taking, and for directing the renovation of the buildings, which freed the team up to heal the patients and to experience the pleasure of working in these amazing buildings.

Dean, my practice manager, for his vision of a happy, driven team and cared-for patients.

Thank you to Nikki Rose, for looking after my magnetic resonance patients. Such a caring, gentle soul, giving patients a lot of her time.

Erica and Jean, who look after patient bookings, man the phones, and look after the needy patients in reception with compassion.

My business consultant, Lesley Bruce, thank you for listening to my woes, and for your time and passion about management strategies and patient care.

My IT consultant, Lee Marsh, thank you for all our incredible IT.

My web designer, Chris, for helping Alan with websites, and also Tom Price, thank you.

My creative designer, Simon, for helping me with great logos and artwork.

My marketing consultant and social media advisor, Eleanor Piredda, new to our team and so inspiring and hardworking.

My gardener to the clinic grounds, Chris. Your flowers and landscaping inspires my patients.

The ladies at 'Help At Hand' who help with the cleaning.

Andy Lewis, I appreciate your hard work in creating a new writing and painting room at my house, as well as your building work at the clinics and on my greenhouse.

My presenting life:

Professor Gunn, thank you for all your many hours of teaching in London, Vancouver, and Korea. It is such an honour to lecture alongside you and to receive the honorary fellowship.

Joseph McClendon, it is always a mixture of nerves and excitement co-presenting with you. You and Tony Robbins are truly mind-bendingly inspirational.

Fasila, thanks for event managing and great tea breaks.

John Parker, a delight to present with, and I listen to your CD on meditation a lot.

Goedele Leyssen, I can't wait to read your yoga book, *Boost*, once it is out in English.

Ronnie Ruiz, my Mr Water knowledge man, thank you.

Jon Hobbs, it was a privilege to meet you and discuss theories with such a passionate, hardworking lecturer, and I look forward to working with you in book two.

Mr Bandler, thank you for your teachings on NLP and stage fright.

Jess Coleman, my editor, so patient and her attention to detail is incredible.

Ruth Fry, for the arduous task of the exercise sketches.

Alex Styles Photography, for being wonderful at putting me at ease.

Penny Grimley, my makeup artist for the shoot.

Shirley Harvey Bates, watercolour artist in Montreal, truly a genius.

Tanya Back, for typesetting this book.

Tim Rumbelow, for doing my video interviewing. Such an enthusiast.

Appendix

Questionnaires

Throughout the book, I've put reminders to fill in these questionnaires in order to see where you rate in terms of mindset, nutrition and hydration, fitness, and lifestyle. This is my traffic light approach to health, and your answers will determine whether you are in the green category (good), the amber category (room for improvement) or the red category (poor). These are your fitness keys, and they will tell you which areas you need to focus on. Once you've read the chapters and started making changes in your life, take the questionnaire again and see how much you have improved.

Questionnaire for Mindset

Do you regularly indulge in the following activities in order to improve your mindset?

• Practise tai chi / yoga / stretching / gentle pilates?	YES	NO
• Meditate / pray / sit quietly / study NLP?	YES	NO
• Have a massage / reiki / acupuncture / reflexology?	YES	NO
• Relax outside in the countryside / by the sea with gardening / reading / walking?	YES	NO
• Have a hobby with artistic expression e.g. music / painting pictures?	YES	NO
• Restrict TV time to useful, pleasant viewing?	YES	NO
• Listen to your favourite music regularly?	YES	NO
• Regularly talk over any worries with a close family member of friend?	YES	NO
• Have meaningful relationships at work and home?	YES	NO

---

0 – 3: RED.

3 – 6: AMBER.

6 – 9: GREEN.

Scores: Now count up your scores – are you red, amber, or green for this key?

Initial score:

Once you've read the chapter and implemented any changes, take the questionnaire again to see how much you've improved.

Secondary score:

Questionnaire for Nutrition and Hydration

This questionnaire is in four parts.

Diet and Blood Sugar Levels

- Is your weight good for your age and height?   YES   NO
- Do you have lots of energy and do you like to exercise?   YES   NO
- Are you free from joint pain?   YES   NO
- Do you rarely feel like dozing in the day and feel alert after eating?   YES   NO
- Do you hardly ever get stomach ache or bloating?   YES   NO
- Do you concentrate easily with a clear memory and few headaches?   YES   NO
- Do you hardly ever need sweet food or caffeine fixes?   YES   NO
- Do you jump out of bed, raring to go?   YES   NO
- Do you rarely feel dizzy / irritable / have mood swings in gaps between meals?   YES   NO

Water

- Do you rarely have thirst / dry mouth?   YES   NO
- Do you rarely get headaches?   YES   NO
- Is your urine a mild (not dark) yellow colour?   YES   NO
- Are your skin and lips moist, not dry?   YES   NO
- Do you have regular bowel movements most days?   YES   NO
- Do you have less than two glasses of alcohol a day?   YES   NO
- Do you have five helpings of fresh fruit and vegetables a day?   YES   NO
- Do you have several glasses of fruit water / juice / herbal teas a day, even if resting?   YES   NO
- Do you avoid having too many salty snacks?   YES   NO

Healthy Low Homocysteine Levels (repairing DNA and building nerves / cartilage)

- Is your weight satisfactory and stable?   YES   NO
- Are you a clear thinker with a good memory and rare headaches?   YES   NO
- Do you eat healthily with green veggies, seeds, and nuts, but aren't vegan?   YES   NO

- You are not an alcoholic, smoker, or heavy coffee drinker? YES NO
- Do you have little joint pain? YES NO
- Do you have great stamina without weariness? YES NO
- Is your cardiovascular system and blood pressure normal? YES NO
- Do you sleep well? YES NO
- Are you rarely angry, irritable, or down? YES NO

Essential Fats

- Do you have healthy hair? YES NO
- Do you have flexible, pain-free joints? YES NO
- You are not taking painkillers? YES NO
- No arthritis, asthma, or eczema? YES NO
- No diagnosed cardiovascular problems? YES NO
- Do you spend more than thirty minutes a day outside in sunlight? YES NO
- Do you eat healthily with oily fish, about four eggs a week, seeds and nuts most days, and fewer than two alcoholic drinks a day? YES NO
- Do you have a good memory, learning abilities, and concentration? YES NO
- You don't get down, anxious or unnecessarily angry? YES NO

Anti-Ageing, Anti-rot, Antioxidants

- Are you a quick healer? YES NO
- Are you younger than middle aged (40)? YES NO
- Do you have healthy skin? YES NO
- No diagnosis of cancer or cardiovascular disease? YES NO
- Don't bruise easily? YES NO
- Do you live in quiet, clear air, healthy countryside, not near major roads? YES NO
- Do you eat healthily with five lots of fruit and veg a day, raw seeds / nuts, and at least two oily fish a week? YES NO
- Do you take antioxidant supplements? YES NO
- Do you exercise and raise your heart rate five times a week? YES NO

0 – 3: RED.

3 – 6: AMBER.

6 – 9: GREEN.

Scores: Now count up your scores – are you red, amber, or green for this key?

Initial score:

Once you've read the chapter and implemented any changes, take the questionnaire again to see how much you've improved.

Secondary score:

Questionnaire for Fitness

Looking at Exercise

• Do you do some form of exercise every day for at least half an hour?	YES	NO
• Do you exercise to raise your heart beat with aerobic exercise for at least half an hour, two or three times a week?	YES	NO
• Do you have a physical / manual job that restricts sitting time?	YES	NO
• Could you run if you had to?	YES	NO
• Do you get in and out of the car easily and climb stairs without pain?	YES	NO
• Do you regularly swim / gym / play golf / play football etc.?	YES	NO
• Can you touch your toes and lift your legs and arms up easily without pain?	YES	NO
• Do you stretch regularly with relative ease?	YES	NO
• Do you strengthen your body regularly through weights at the gym or work?	YES	NO

---

0 – 3: RED.

3 – 6: AMBER.

6 – 9: GREEN.

Scores: Now count up your scores – are you red, amber, or green for this key?

Initial score:

Once you've read the chapter and implemented any changes, take the questionnaire again to see how much you've improved.

Secondary score:

Questionnaire for Lifestyle

Do you take measures to control your stress levels?

- Do you enjoy your career and restrict the hours you work? YES NO
- Do you drive stress-free, short distances every day in locations you like? YES NO
- Do you spend enough time relaxing before bed and sleep well? YES NO
- Do you enjoy a peaceful, loving home life with a fit, well family and fit pets? YES NO
- Do you have few money worries? YES NO
- Do you enjoy and can take holidays as you feel you need them? YES NO
- Do you have a strong purpose to life and achieve enjoyable goals? YES NO
- Do you not depend on alcohol / sweets / unhealthy food to calm you? YES NO
- Do you enjoy living where you are in a healthy, attractive, peaceful environment? YES NO

---

0 – 3: RED.
3 – 6: AMBER.
6 – 9: GREEN.
Scores: Now count up your scores – are you red, amber, or green for this key?

Initial score:

Once you've read the chapter and implemented any changes, take the questionnaire again to see how much you've improved.

Secondary score:

List of Angels

- **Melchisadec:** father of angels of the divine presence, rainbow and violet ray, mind body soul union.
- **Raphael:** my youngest nephew's namesake, angel of mercury, summoned if stressed, or going through upheaval and travel. I have a lovely picture floating though heaven with babies in the angel's arms. Patron angel of healers, works with the immune system, and candles depict a golden yellow ray.
- **Caduceus:** healing symbol.
- **Ariel:** also an angel of healing, especially with reiki, and with lungs and throat issues.
- **Uriel:** angel of fire and alchemy, the planet Uranus, freedom, creativity and transformation, something that I treasure for myself and my patients. Erasing old patterns of behaviour with an orange yellow flame. Creating a brighter future by freeing you from your past.
- **Cassiel:** is about opposites being necessary – without darkness we cannot appreciate light, and about our attitude to a difficulty, he helps us with suffering and finding our true direction back to how we should be.
- **Michael:** protector, warrior against darkness, angel of the sun.
- **Gabriel:** angel of the moon and integrating feminine wisdom with masculine to know thyself and others.
- **Camael:** when bruised and battered by circumstance, crimson/red ray.
- **Sandalphon:** angel of prayer, he carries your prayers to the creator, feathers are symbolic.
- **Sahaqiel:** angel of the sky.
- **Raziel:** records all earthly and celestial knowledge, guiding Adam, Enoch, and Solomon, and guiding Noah to rebuild the world after the floods. New learning is needed to get out of a rut when you call on this angel. A new learning adventure to share with others.
- **Haniel:** angel of love, for all those dear to you and the planet and universe, unconditional love.
- **Phuel:** angel of the waters and moon. Calming emotions.
- **Zadkiel:** abundance associated with kindness, highest good, and harm none.

- **Hermes Trismegistus:** angel of spiritual alchemy, teaching God given will of three, as in Holy trinity and mind body spirit, psychically work for highest good.
- **Metatron:** God in man.
- **Shekinah:** God in woman, guardians of the tree of life, ten roots and guiding humans back to the creature.
- **Rachmiel:** compassion and caring, who soothes the sick humans and animals.
- **Hariel:** arts, sciences, and especially tame animals.
- **Tubiel:** birds.
- **Achaiah:** angel of connection with the planet and giving thanks to nature.
- **Sachluph:** plants.
- **Isda:** food and nourishment for health and physical wholeness.
- **Zeruch:** strength.
- **Phanuel:** atonement, both prayed to at times of matters of the heart and dark issues.
- **Tabris:** free will.
- **Oriel:** destiny, they are about free will and decisions, and talk of the choices of fallen angels.
- **Radueriel:** arts, poetry, and music.
- **Manakel:** of aquatic creatures.

There are twelve zodiac angels, and mine is Zuriel, as I'm a Libra, wanting harmony, being indecisive, endlessly weighing up pros and cons, and avoiding disharmony to the detriment of happiness. Pistis Sophia is the mother of the zodiac angels and has heavenly wisdom. She is also called Quan Yin, Mother Mary, and Eve. She wants you to be true to your divine template.

Health Hub and Nutritional Tests

Patrick Holford has been recognised as an authority on nutrition for many years, and he has developed a comprehensive health check questionnaire which has already been completed by over 55,000 people. For more information, take a look at www.patrickholford.com.

YorkTest

Modern lifestyles have led to an explosion of obesity, diabetes, heart conditions, cancer, and osteoarthritis, to name just a few. Obesity, diabetes, and liver damage are all closely linked to glycaemic load and this can be measured with a blood test at the clinic. The analysis is then done at YorkTest (www.yorktest.com), and a liver check test is also available.

Homocysteine can similarly be analysed. Most people in the UK have never heard of homocysteine and are unaware that it is the most important predictor of many degenerative diseases, such as heart disease, strokes, and peripheral artery disease. A homocysteine level above 13 has been shown to predict 67% of all deaths within five years. A quick blood test is all that is needed for you to find out how much at risk you are.

Around 45% of UK residents suffer from some form of food intolerance, which can manifest itself either rapidly – such as with a peanut allergy – or more slowly, with symptoms such as IBS, pain after eating, eczema, or asthma. A comprehensive food intolerance test is available, which will analyse your tolerance on the YorkTest website.

Vitamins – Antioxidants

When I need vitamins and minerals, I use USANA Health Sciences (www.usana.com), a USA company. I've been taking them for years, ever since reading research on the top 500 companies in North America – USANA came up trumps.

These should include vitamins A, E, C and B, carotene/retinol, zinc, selenium, glutathione, cysteine, anthocyanins of berry extract, lipoic acid, and coenzyme Q10.

Minerals

Useful minerals include calcium, magnesium, boron, zinc, silica, and many more. I currently take USANA essentials.

Digestive Enzymes and Support

Patrick Holford uses BioCare probiotics, and I had some when my stress levels were a little high; it was prescribed to me by an in-house nutritionist at the clinic. I am currently being introduced to Nature's Sunshine Products, and some of them look very good. However, ideally, I still like an expert on board if recommending to patients.

Mind Nutrients

If you were to look in my cupboard at home, you'd find BioCare, Patrick Holford's Mood Food, TMG, 5-HTP, chromium complex, B vitamins, brain food, and contact formulae, also containing TMG (a homocysteine regulator).

Essential Fats and Fish Oils

Look for omega 3, DHA, EPA, and GLA, which is omega 6. Also, BioCare essential omegas and Seven Seas cod liver oil.

Joint Care

Personally, I use USANA Health Science's Procosa II, but you can also use vitamin C, manganese, glucosamine sulphate, turmeric, silica, BioCare joint support, glucosamine hydrochloride, MSM, hops, olives, curcumin, quercetin, Solgar Gold, DLPA, and niacin.

Exercises

Pic#	Picture	Exercise Name	Pg#
1		Arm exercise biceps with weights.	147
2		Butterfly stretch for inner thigh.	177
3		Abdominal breath for core set.	182
4		Cat back stretch.	176
5		Knee hugs to curl up spine.	153
6		Stability core work for lumbar spine.	122
7		Hamstring exercise with weights.	148
8		Quads exercise with weights.	149
9		Single knee hug, stretches hip.	153
10		Rest position/child pose to stretch spine.	152

Pic#	Picture	Exercise Name	Pg#
11		Post legmuscle hamstring stretch.	154
12		Abduction outer hip exercise with weight.	149
13		Running.	116
14		Adductor inner hip exercise with weight.	150
15		Corkscrew shoulder stability exercise, also qi kong bird arm.	173
16		Fitball with leg stability drill.	167
17		Fitball with good posture and pelvic stability drill.	120
18		Fitball bridge exercise.	168
19		Chi kong.	173
20		Chi kong.	173
21		Dumb waiter.	152

Pic#	Picture	Exercise Name	Pg#
22		Standing pose legs together.	171
23		Tai chi standing pose knees soft.	171
24		Head to knees forward bend on floor.	178
25		Triceps with weights.	147
26		Reach up to sky standing pose.	179
27		Cobra back stretch.	176
28		Bridging back or roll down.	121
29		Dead bug back stability exercise.	123
30		Superman.	122
31		Pecs exercise with weights.	148
32		Biceps with weights, different angle.	147

Pic#	Picture	Exercise Name	Pg#
33		Strengthening shoulder lateral rotator muscles.	149
34		Stretching inner thigh adductors.	155
35		Stretching out thigh muscles, quads and hip flexors.	153
36		Stretching out hips in sitting position.	178
37		Yoga sitting position.	182
38		Knee leg rolls.	153
39		Abdominal curl ups.	121
40		Nordic pole walking.	163
41		Warrior pose and calf stretch.	154
42		Forward spine bend.	152
43		Neck stretches.	151

Resources – Health

Deepak Chopra
Books and The Chopra Foundation – www.deepakchopra.com.

E.F.T
Gary Craig's website for free downloads – www.emofree.com.

HeartMath
Products to improve your health – www.heartmath.com.

Jon Hobbs
AACP director, lecturer, and physiotherapist, he currently runs accredited courses in acupuncture for women's health problems – Jon_acupuncture@btinternet.com.

MRT
Magnetic Resonance Treatment centre in Staffordshire – www.mrtcentre.co.uk.

Naturopathic information
Pam Cartwright c/o www.painreliefclinic.co.uk.
Jules Cattell – www.equilibria-health.com.

The Pain Relief Clinic
Nicky Snazell's clinic in Staffordshire – www.painreliefclinic.co.uk.

The Pain Killer
Nicky Snazell (author) – www.thepainkiller.co.uk.

Patrick Holford
Courses and health club – www.patrickholford.com.

Photography
Alex Styles – www.alexstyles.co.uk.

Tony Robbins
UPW seminars and coaching – www.tonyrobbins.com.

The Z Factor
Joseph McClendon seminar co-starring guess who?! – www.z-factor.net.

Resources – Book

Editor

Book Editing – Jessica Coleman – www.colemanediting.co.uk.

Exercise Illustrations

Ruth Fry – ruth.le.fry@googlemail.com.

Makeup Artist

For photo shoot – Penny Grimley – www.pennygrimley.com.

Marketing

Eleanor Piredda – Epiredda@marketingsense.co.uk.

Typesetting

Tanya Back – www.tanyabackdesigns.com.

Watercolour Artist

Shirley Harvey Bates – shirleyharveybates@gmail.com.

Bibliography

Mindset

Bandler, Richard Dr. *How To Take Charge Of Your Life*. HarperCollins, 2014.

Bandler, Richard Dr. *Magic In Action*. Meta Publications, 1992.

Bandler, Richard Dr. *Make Your Life Great*. HarperCollins, 2008.

Bandler, Richard Dr. and Fitzpatrick, Owen. *Conversations*. Mysterious Publications, 2009.

Bandler, Richard Dr. and Grinder, John. *Frogs Into Princes*.

Bandler, Richard Dr. and La Valle, John. Persuasion Engineering. Meta Publications Inc, 1996.

Bandler, Richard Dr. and Thomson, Garner. *The Secrets Of Being Happy*. IM Press, 2001.

Bays, Brandon and Billett, Kevin. *The Journey – Consciousness The New Currency*. Weidenfeld and Nicolson, 2002.

Browne, Sylvia. *Temples On The Other Side*. Hay House, 2008.

Buckland, Raymond. *Practical Candleburning Rituals*. Llewellyn Publications, 2013.

Buzan, Tony. *The Power Of Spiritual Intelligence*. HarperCollins, 2001.

Byrne, Rhonda. *The Power*. Simon And Schuster UK Ltd, 2010.

Carter, Rita. *Consciousness*. Weidenfeld and Nicolson, 2002.

Carter, Rita. *Mapping The Mind*. Phoenix, 2010.

Carter, Rita. *Multiplicity: The New Science Of Personality*. Little, Brown, 2008.

Chopra, Deepak Dr. *Perfect Health*. Bantam Books, 2001. Real People Press, 1979.

Chopra, Deepak Dr. *Reinventing The Body, Resurrecting The Soul*. Rider, 2009.

Chopra, Deepak Dr. *The Book Of Secrets*. Rider, 2004.

Chopra, Deepak Dr. *The Third Jesus*. Rider, 2008.

Chopra, Deepak Dr. *The Way Of The Wizard*. Ebury Publishing, 2000.

Chopra, Deepak Dr. *Unconditional Life*. Bantam Books, 1991.

Cole, Frances Dr, Macdonald H, Carus, C and Howden-Leach H. *Overcoming Chronic Pain*. Robinson, 2010.

Cross, John. *Healing With The Chakra Energy System*. North Atlantic Books, 2006.

Cunningham, Scott. *Magical Aromatherapy*. Llewellyn Publications, 2013.

Dyer, Wayne Dr. *A New Way Of Thinking, A New Way Of Being*. Hay House UK, 2010.

Dyer, Wayne Dr. *Change Your Thoughts Change Your Life*. Hay House, 2010.

Dyer, Wayne Dr. *Wisdom Of The Ages*. Thorsons, 1998.

Eden, Donna and Dahlin, Dondi. *The Little Book Of Energy Medicine*. Penguin Group, 2012.

Edwards, Gill. *Conscious Medicine*. Piatkus, 2010.

Epstein, Donald M Dr. *The 12 Stages Of Healing*. New World Library, 1994.

Coelho, Paulo. *Manual Of The Light Worker*. HarperCollins, 2003.

Goleman, Daniel Dr. *Social Intelligence*. Hutchinson, 2006.

Gunn, Chan. *The Gunn Approach To The Treatment Of Chronic Pain*. Churchill Livingstone, 2003.

Hanscom, David Dr. *Back In Control*. Vertus Press, 2012.

Harding, Jennie. *Incense*. Cambridge University Press, 2005.

Heaven, Ross. *The Journey To You*. Bantam Books, 2001.

Hewitt, William. *Hypnosis For Beginners*. Llewellyn Publications, 2005.

Hill, Napoleon. *Think And Grow Rich*. Wilder Publications, 2007.

Holford, Patrick. *Beat Stress And Fatigue*. Piatkus, 1999.

Holford, Patrick. *The Feel Good Factor*. Piatkus, 2011.

James, Tad, Shephard, David, Flores, Lorraine and Schober, Jack. *Hypnosis*. Crown House Publishing Ltd, 2005.

Lee, John R. *What Your Doctor May Not Tell You About Premenopause*. Warner, 1999.

Levine, Peter. *Waking The Tiger*. North Atlantic Books Publishers, 1997.

Loyd, Alex and Johnson, Ben. *The Healing Code*. Intermedia Publishing Group, 2010.

McClendon, Joseph. *Get Happy NOW!* Success Books, 2012.

Morgan, Marlo. *Mutant Message Down Under*. Thorsons, 1994.

Myss, Carolyn Dr. *Why People Don't Heal And How They Can*. Bantam, 1998.

Naparstek, Belleruth. *Invisible Heroes*. Bantam Books, 2006.

Newton, Michael Dr. *Life Between Lives: Hypnotherapy For Spiritual Regression*. Llewellyn Publications, 2004.

Noble Knight, Jane. *The Inspiring Journeys Of Women Entrepreneurs*. Noble Knight Publishing, 2013.

Northrup, Christiane Dr. *Women's Bodies, Women's Wisdom*. Piatkus, 1998.

O'Connor, Dermot. *The Healing Code*. Hodder Paperbacks, 2006.

Ortner, Nick. *The Tapping Solution (DVD)*.

Perlmutter, David Dr. and Villoldo, Alerberto Dr. *Power Up Your Brain*. Hay House, 2011.

Phillips, Maggie. *Finding The Energy To Heal*. By The Way Publishing Services, 2000.

Phillips, Maggie. *Reversing Chronic Pain*. North Atlantic Books, 2007.

Redfield, James. *The Celestine Prophecy*. Bantam, 1994.

Renault, Dennis and Freke, Timothy. *Principles Of – Native American Spirituality*. HarperCollins, 1996.

Robbins, Anthony. *Awaken The Giant Within*. Pocket Books, 2001.

Rohn, Jim. *Seven Strategies For Wealth And Happiness*. Three Rivers Press, 1996.

Sadler, Jan. *Pain Relief Without Drugs*. Element Books, 2007.

Sarno, John Dr. *Healing Back Pain*. Wellness Central, 1991.

Sarno, John Dr. *The Mind Body Prescription*. Hatchett Book Group, 1998.

Schultz, Mona Lisa Dr. *Awakening Intuition*. Transworld Publishers, 1998.

Scott, Ginger. *Scents Of The Soul*. Findhorn Press Ltd, 2009.

Shealy, Norman C Dr. *Energy Medicine*. Dimension Press, 2011.

Shealy, Norman C Dr. *Life Beyond 100*. Penguin Group, 2006.

Shealy, Norman C Dr. *Medical Intuition*. A.R.E Press Publishers, 2010.

Shealy, Norman C Dr. *Soul Medicine*. Energy Psychology Press, 2008.

Siegel, Bernie Dr. *Love, Medicine And Miracles*. Rider, 1986.

Snazell, Nicky. *Staffordshire Life Magazine*. Monthly articles over three years.

Snazell, Nicky. *The Pain Jungle*. Positive Health Journal Issue 111, May 2005.

Stein, Diane. *Essential Reiki*. Crossing Press, 1995.

Thomson, Garner and Khan, Khalid Dr. *Magic In Practice*. Hammersmith Press Ltd, 2008.

Tolle, Eckhart. *Stillness Speaks*. New World Library, 2003.

Van Praagh, James. *Heaven And Earth*. Rider, 2001.

Veltheim, John. *The BodyTalk System*. Parama, 1999.

Villoldo, Alberto Dr. *Dance Of The Four Winds*. HarperCollins, 1995.

Villoldo, Alberto Dr. *Healing States*. Simon And Schuster, Inc, 1987.

Villoldo, Alberto Dr. *Illumination*. Hay House UK, 2010.

Villoldo, Alberto Dr. *Mending The Past And Healing The Future With Soul Retrieval*. Hay House UK, 2005.

Villoldo, Alberto Dr. *Shaman, Healer, Sage*. Bantam Books, 2001.

Villoldo, Alberto Dr. *The Four Insights*. Hay House UK, 2006.

Villoldo, Alberto Dr. and Perlmutter, David Dr. *Power Up Your Brain*. Hay House, 2001.

Walsch, Neale Donald. *When Everything Changes, Change Everything*. Hodder and Stoughton, 2009.

Weiss, Brian Dr. *Only Love Is Real*. Piatkus, 1996.

Weiss, Brian Dr. *Same Soul Different Body*. Piatkus, 2004.

Wentz, Myron. *Invisible Miracles*. Self published, 2002.

Wesselman, Hank Dr. *Spirit Medicine*. Hay House UK, 2004.

Westwood, Christine. *Aromatherapy Stress Management*. Amberwood Publishing Ltd, 1995.

Whang, Sang. *Reverse Aging*. JSP Publishing, 2010.

Wilde, Stuart. *Silent Power*. Hay House, 1996.

Nutrition and Hydration

Allison, M C et al. 1984. 'Gastrointestinal damage associated with the use of non-steroidal anti-inflammatory drugs' *The Lancet*, vol 843(2), pp. 1171-1174.

Baranowski, T and Stables, G 2000. 'Process evaluations of the 5 a day projects' *Health Education And Behaviour*, vol 27(2), pp. 157-166.

Batmanghelidj, F. *Your Body's Many Cries For Water*. GHS Inc., 2008.

British Medical Association. *New Guide To Medicines And Drugs*. Dorling Kindersley Limited, 1994.

Boggs, D A, Palmer, J R, Wise, L A et al. 2010. 'Fruit and veg intake in relation to risk of breast cancer in the black women's health study' *The American Journal Of Epidemiology*, vol 10, p 293).

Cairney, Edward. *The Sprouters Handbook*. Argyll Publishing, 2011.

Chopra, Deepak. *What Are You Hungry For?* Rider, 2013.

Colgan, Michael Dr. *The New Nutrition*. Apple Publishing, 2005.

Cullen, J, Bates, D, Laird, N et al. 1995. 'Incidence of adverse drug events and potential drug events' *The Journal Of The American Medical Association*, vol 274, pp. 29-34.

Emoto, Masaru. *Messages From Water And The Universe*. Hay House, 2010.

Flaws, Bob. *The Tao Of Healthy Eating*. The Blue Poppy Press, 1998.

Fowles, Clell M. *Drugs And Nutrient Depletion*. C.M Fowles, 2003.

Fuhrman, Joel. *Eat To Live*. Little, Brown and Company, 2010.

Fuhrman, Joel. *Super Immunity*. HarperCollins, 2011.

Fuhrman, Joel 2000. 'The global infectious disease threat and its implications for the US' *National Intelligence Council*.

Gallop, Rick. *The GI Diet*. Virgin Books, 2004.

Gey, K F and Alfthan G A 1997. 'Plasma homocysteine and cardiovascular disease mortality.' *The Lancet*, vol 359, p 397.

Glenville, Marilyn. *Fat Around The Middle*. Kyle Cathie Limited, 2006.

Gullet, N P, Ruhul Amin A R 2010. 'Cancer prevention with natural compounds' *Semin Oncol*, vol 37, pp. 258-81.

Hamyln Cookbooks. *200 Juices And Smoothies*. Hamlyn, 2008.

Holford, Patrick. *Good Medicine*. Piatkus, 2014.

Holford, Patrick. *Improve Your Digestion*. Piatkus, 1999.

Holford, Patrick. *Say No To Arthritis*. Piatkus, 2009.

Holford, Patrick. *The 10 Secrets Of 100% Healthy Ageing*. Piatkus, 2009.

Holford, Patrick. *The Optimum Nutrition Bible*. Piatkus, 2009.

Holford, Patrick and Braly, James Dr. *The H Factor*. Piatkus, 2003.

Holford, Patrick and Burne, Jerome. *Food Is Better Medicine Than Drugs*. Piatkus, 2006.

Klepser, T and Klepser, M 1999. 'Unsafe and potentially safe herbal therapies' *American Journal Of American Health*, vol 56, pp. 125-38.

Lazarou, I, Pomeranz, B and Corey, P 1998. 'Incidence of adverse drug events and potential drug events' *The Journal Of The American Medical Association*, vol 279, pp. 1200-05.

Li, C, Ford, ES, Zhao, G. et al 2010. 'Serum alpha-carotene concentrations and risk of death among US adults' 3*rd* *National Health and Nutritional Exam Survey*, vol Nov 22, p 440.

Lichtenstein et al. 2000, *New England Journal Of Medicine*, vol 343(2), pp. 1233-6.

Lu, Henry C. *Chinese System Of Food Cures*. Sterling Publishing Company, 1986.

McKeith, Gillian Dr. *You Are What You Eat*. Penguin Group Publishers, 2004.

Millidge, Judith. *Smoothies And Juicing*. Silverdale Books, 2002.

Moldoveanu, B 2008. 'Inflammatory mechanisms in the lung' *Journal Of Inflammation Research*, vol 2009:2, pp. 1 – 11.

Patten, M. and Ewin, J. *Eat To Beat Arthritis*. Thorsons, 2004.

Patterson, Rachel. *Kitchen Witchcraft*. Moon Books, 2013.

Reginster, J Y et al. 2001. 'Long-term effects of glucosamine sulphate on osteoarthritis progression; a randomised, placebo controlled clinical trial' *The Lancet*, vol 357, pp. 251-256.

Rose, Natalia. *The Raw Food Detox Diet*. HarperCollins, 2005.

Roundtree, R 1999. 'Herbs and drugs for your heart; sorting out what's safe' *Herbs for Health*, Nov/Dec 1999, pp. 28-29.

Segnit, Niki. *The Flavour Thesaurus*. Bloomsbury, 2010.

Stiles, Tara. *Make Your Own Rules Diet*. Hay House UK, 2014.

Strand, Ray D. *Death By Prescription*. Thomas Nelson Publishers, 2003.

Strand, Ray D. *Health For Life*. Real Life Press, 2005.

Strand, Ray D. *Healthy For Life*. Real Life Press, 2004.

Vale, Jason. *The Juice Master*, 2005.

Vyas, Bharti and Le Quesne, S. *The Ph Diet*. Thorsons, 2004.

Waterland, R A and Jirtle, R J, 2003. *Molecular And Cellular Biology*, vol 23, pp. 5293-5300.

Weindruch, Dr and Sohal, Dr 1997. 'Caloric intake and aging' *The New England Journal Of Medicine*, vol 337(14), pp. 986-94.

Wheater, Caroline. *Juicing For Health*. Thorsons, 2001.

Willcox, B J, Willcox ,D C, Suzuki, M, Todoriki, H 2000. 'Homocysteine levels in Okinawan Japanese' *Journal Of Investigative Medicine*, vol 48(2), p. 205.

Wills, Judith. *The Food Bible*. Quadrille Publishing Limited, 2002.

Young, Robert Dr. and Redford Young, Shelley. *The Ph Miracle: Balance Your Diet, Reclaim Your Health*. Time Warner Books, 2010.

Young, Robert Dr. and Redford Young, Shelley. *The Ph Miracle For Weight Loss*. Time Warner Books, 2006.

Fitness

Collins, Jane. *Ten Minutes To Better Health*. Reader's Digest, 1999.

Dregan, A and Gulliford, M C 2013. 'Leisure-time physical activity over the life course and cognitive functioning in late mid-adult years: a cohort-based investigation' *Psychological Medicine*, vol 43, no. 11, pp. 2447-2458.

Gordon, Debra and Harrar, Sari. *Full Life Repair Kit*. Reader's Digest, 2009.

Kessenich, C R. 1998. 'Tai chi as a method of fall prevention in the elderly' *Orthopaedic Nursing*, vol 17, pp. 27-29.

Kiew Kit, Wong. *Chi Kung For Health And Vitality*. Vermilion, 2001.

Lai, J S, Lan, C, Wong, M K et al. 1995. 'Two year trends in cardiorespiratory function among older tai chi chuan pracitioners and sedentary subjects' *Journal Of The American Geriatrics Society*, vol 43(11), pp. 1222-7.

Lamb, David R. *Physiology Of Exercise*. Macmillan Publishing Company, 1984.

Lan, C, Lai, S, Chen, Y et al. 1998. '12 month tai chi training in the elderly; its effect on health and fitness' *Medicine & Science In Sports & Exercise*, vol 30, pp. 345-351.

Lane, J M and Nydick, M 1999. 'Osteoporosis: current modes of prevention and treatment' *The Journal Of The American Medical Association*, vol 7, pp. 19-31.

Lingpa, Tashi. *Kundalini Yoga*. Kindle Edition, 2014.

McArdle, W, Katch, F and Katch, V. *Exercise Physiology*. Lea and Febiger Publishers, 1991.

McAtee, Robert E. and Charland, Jeff. *Facilitated Stretching*. Human Kinetics Europe Ltd, 2007.

Norris, Chris M. *Abdominal Training*. A and C Black Publishers Ltd, 1997.

Paulson, G. L. *Kundalini And The Chakras*. Llewellyn Publishers, 2005.

Roberts, Matt. *Fitness For Life*. Dorling Kindersley Limited, 2002.

Robinson, Lynne and Convy, Gerry. *The Balanced Workout*. Pan Books, 2000.

Robinson, Lynne, Fisher, Helge, Knox, Jacqueline and Thomson, Gordon. *The Official Body Control Pilates Manual*. Pan Books, 2002.

Robinson, Lynne and Thomson, Gordon. *Body Control*. Pan Books, 1998.

Saltin, Bengt 1966. 'The 1966 bed rest and training study' *Circulation*.

Stiles, Tara. *Yoga Cures*. Three Rivers Press, 2012.

Wolfson, L, Whipple, R, Derby, C et al. 1996. 'Balance and strength training in older adults; intervention gains and tai chi maintenance' *The Journal Of The American Geriatrics Society*, vol 44, pp. 498-506).

Yocum, D, Castrol, L, Corne, M 2000. 'Exercise, education and behavioral modification as alternative therapy for pain and stress' *Rheumatic Disease Clinics Of North America*, vol 26(1), pp. 145-159.

Lifestyle

Bailey, Alice A. *A Treatise On White Magic*. Lucis Press Ltd, 1970.

Bartlett, Richard. *Matrix Energetics*. Beyond Words Publishing, 2007.

Bourgault, Luc. *The American Indian Secrets Of Crystal Healing*. W Foulsham & Co Ltd, 2012.

Buzan, Tony. *The Power Of Creative Intelligence*. HarperCollins, 2001.

Church, Dawson. *The Genie In Your Genes*. Cygnus Books, 2007.

Clogstoun-Willmott, Jonathan. *Stress From Qi Stagnation – Signs Of Stress*. Frame Of Mind Publishing, 2013.

Dawson, Karl and Marillat, Kate. *Transform Your Beliefs, Transform Your Life: EFT Tapping Using Matrix Imprinting*. Hay House UK, 2014.

Dyer, Wayne. *Stop The Excuses*. Hay House UK, 2009.

Frankl, Viktor E. *Man's Search For Meaning*. Rider, 2004.

Goleman, Daniel. *Destructive Emotions: A Scientific Dialogue With The Dalai Lama*. Bantam Books, 2003.

Goleman, Daniel. *Working With Emotional Intelligence*. Bloomsbury Publishing, 1989.

Hale, Gill. *Feng Shui*. Anness Publishing Ltd, 2004.

Haviland-Jones, J, Rosario, H, Wilson, P, and McGuire, T 2005. 'An environmental approach to positive emotion: Flowers' *Evolutionary Psychology*, vol 3, pp. 104-132.

Heaven, Ross. *Spirit In The City*. Transworld Publishers, 2002.

Keown, Daniel Dr. *The Spark In The Machine*. Singing Dragon, 2014.

Lilly, Sue. *The Magic Of Crystals – Colour And Chakra*. Hermes House, 2011.

Lipton, Bruce. *The Biology Of Belief*. Cygnus Book Publishers, 2005.

Murphy-Hiscock, Arin. *Solitary Wicca For Life*. Adams Media Corporation, 2005.

Myss, Caroline. *Sacred Contracts*. Harmony Books Publishers, 2002.

Noble Knight, Jane. *The Inspiring Journeys Of Women Entrepreneurs*. Noble Knight Publishing UK, 2013.

Robbins, Anthony. and McClendon, Joseph. *Unlimited Power: A Black Choice*. Fireside, 1997.

Roberts, Llyn and Levy, Robert. *Shamanic Reiki*. Moon Books, 2008.

Shealy, Norman and Church, Dawson. *Soul Medicine*. Bang Printing, 2008.

Sulzberger, Robert. *Cottage Gardens*. Aura Books Publishers, 2002.

Usui, Mikao. *The Original Reiki Handbook*. Lotus Press, 1994.

Warner, Felicity. *The Soul Midwives' Handbook*. Hay House UK, 2013.

Weatherup, Katie. *Sacred Travel – Practical Shamanism For Your Vacations And Vision Quests*. Hands Over Heart, 2013.

Willcox, Bradley, Willcox, Craig and Suzuki, Makoto. *The Okinawa Way*. The Penguin Group, 1996.

Worwood, Valerie Ann. *The Fragrant Pharmacy*. Macmillan London Ltd Publishers, 1991.

Wyer, Carol. *Grumpy Old Menopause*. Safkhet Select, 2013.

Introduction to
The Human Garage,
Nicky Snazell's next book.

My team of friends come to work at my practice armed with their nursing, physiotherapy, sports therapy, and orthopaedic surgical medical degrees. Also, for some of them, reiki training, as they are both mechanics and healers.

Once here, they start studying and applying my integrative approach, as so often we seem to work in the illness industry, not the wellness industry. In my clinics, we utilise all the hard work that researchers have put in to be able to create the latest technology – for example, those who scientifically measure how healthy our cells are. Take Quadscan, for instance, that we use for cellular health analysis, measuring nutrients, fat, water, bone, and muscle ratios. Heartmath can be used for measuring heart rate variance (HRV), as well as evaluating mindset and the ability to create the correct mind state for healing – and not stressing. We can assess fitness, how well our lungs and heart cope with exercise, and how flexible and strong we are. Where pressure moves up through our feet and body as we run and walk, we can use gait scanning and biomechanical assessment, looking at how we can improve our posture and reduce joint wear.

Then we carry out physiotherapy and neuropathic pain detailed assessments and prescribe tailor-made treatment plans with mind state and nutrition advice, massage, manipulation, acupuncture, revolutionary IMS for nerve pain, exercise prescription for life, and electrotherapy such as shockwave, laser, and ultrasound. Then, once we are happy that we have got the patient as close to optimum health as is now possible for them, we integrate with revolutionary technology: magnetic resonance (MRT) that pushes back the hands of time. That's right – never before have we had the capability at our fingertips to regrow cartilage and bone cells at an accelerated rate, which normally would not regenerate at all due to ageing. Never before have we gone this far within physical medicine. Star trek-like technology is slowly emerging as the new science of today, and most importantly, it allows us to be more accepting of the mind-body link.

With my background, I am very aware of the power of the mind and I feel privileged to be in the driving seat of the physical medicine of tomorrow. I strongly feel that analysing any block to a patient getting the healing results they want is incredibly important. Keeping accurate records and applying both an intuitive and scientific approach will give a broader understanding, as we are paving the way forward for healing future generations.

Throughout my second book, I am going to share with you my recipes of integrated medicine for physical health. Through sharing with you true stories of just a handful of my current patients (the stories are a composite to disguise them and protect their privacy), my aim is to get you to be able to walk in their shoes, feel their pain, and hear their stories and beliefs about suffering so you can then relate it to your own. Only through getting those light bulb moments – those ah ah's! – are you in a good place to heal. I want to open up an awareness in you about the stories you tell yourself and how self-destructive they can be. A lady said to me only this week, "if my suffering helps another soul, then I can bear it more easily".

My patients are too shy to be on stage, so when I do live shows, I came up with the idea of having puppets made and dressing them up to represent them, allowing me to carry these troubled souls into this room for you.

Have you got hidden beliefs/tragic memories locked into a place in your body? Then let me help you with them.

We all tell ourselves a story – I know I do – for every injury or operation we have, and I have to be careful how I replay my story, as memory is fluid and every time we recall one, we mould a new version of it.

So, let's rewrite your story about your life, starting today.